Our Food Dilemma

Dear Rachel:

A beauty from our 516
and you represent her very
well!

Sincerely,
DT

Our Food Dilemma

Dangerous Foods, Junk Foods, and Superfoods
Do You Know Which Is Which And Why

Dr. Frank J Trapani

To order additional copies, please contact us.
BookSurge, LLC
www.booksurge.com
1-866-308-6235
orders@booksurge.com

Our Food Dilemma

TABLE OF CONTENTS

Acknowledgements

Without certain people this book might never have been written. The first and most important was my father Paul Trapani. Early in our family life he led our family into healthy living. When all of my friends were eating lunches made with white bread, we were made to eat whole wheat. Only brown rice could be found on our table, never white polished and always fresh vegetables and fruit. While many of our friends smoked we were admonished of its dangers. This was long before it became common knowledge that it caused cancer and emphysema. Dad was an architect, but spent many hours studying and learning about health. His interest in health began many years before I was even born

His mentor was a man named Bernarr McFadden. In our home we had a health encyclopedia published by Mr. McFadden as well as his health magazines, which Dad referred to many times. McFadden's story was very fascinating. He was from a rather well to do family, but living at the turn of the century, he contracted tuberculosis at a very early age. His family well able to afford it sent him to a health sanatorium in Switzerland. At that sanatorium he learned the benefits of fresh air, fresh fruits and vegetables and unrefined food. In that manner he was cured. McFadden brought those natural methods back to the U.S. and was the "father" of what came to be known as "The Natural Health Movement" here in America. With those basics applied to our family I can honestly say that we were seldom sick. But, this was many years ago. I owe a lot to Dad for whetting my appetite to learn more about health.

It is interesting to note that Bernarr McFadden had a very serious follower named Paul Bragg. I'm proud to say that Paul and I met and became good friends when we both lived in Hawaii. I consider the late Paul Bragg to have been one of my most important mentors. He was an author/ lecture like none other, and was a great inspiration to me.

While living in Hawaii we became involved with an organization called The National Health Federation. Our "Hui Olo Kino chapter was responsible for organizing conventions there. In doing so we had the opportunity to meet and learn from those many personalities in the Natural health field. Betty Lee Morales, Bob Hoffman, and Adele Davis, just to mention a few. These are a few of the many people to whom I owe a lot.

With that said I must mention here my wife Sonia and her mother Sofia. Like my father, Sofia had an innate wisdom for good health, which Sonia brought into our relationship. It all made good sense to us and we brought our children up accordingly. I'm sure you would laugh at some of the stories we could tell about the food my wife prepared for our children. But it is a fact that we were never up a single night with a sick child! Our son Stephen is a chiropractor like his dad and our two daughters, while not in the health field are bringing up their children in the same manner and with the same results.

In fact, it was my both daughters Lisa and Eva who have been after me for years to write this book. So, My Dears. Here it is!

Finally, thanks to my editor Candace Rose who patiently corrected all of my grammatical errors.

Zorba: Why do the young die? Why does anyone die? can you tell me?

Young Englishman: I don't know!

Zorba: (angrily) What good are all your d-mn books, if they don't tell you that,
what the h-ll do they tell you?

Young Englishman: They tell me of the agony of men who can't
answer questions like yours.

Zorba the Greek – A novel by Nikos Kazantzakis.

To my Father, Paul Trapani

1.

Introduction

Why do people die? You've heard it said that this person or that person died of "old age" Were their bodies uniformly 'worn out ? Did they succumb to some illness? Did they die from a specific disease, or did just one organ "fail"?

It could be cancer, heart disease, kidney failure, liver disease, immune system failure or a host of other pathologies. But in most cases, the remainder of the organs in those individuals are unaffected. Many of those "bodies" could still be functional, were it not for that specific failed organ. It's almost like saying that if our car battery goes bad, we should junk the entire car. Or, if a hose on the washing machine breaks, the whole machine must be discarded.

When one dies, we must ask the question "why"? Surely our genes and environment must have something to do with it, and indeed, they do!

Yet I have always functioned under the assumption and belief that at least 90% of all illness and disease can be related to our dietary habits one way or another. By that I mean our health is determined by both deficiencies of nutrients (omissions) as well as by those things that shouldn't come into our bodies, but do (commissions).

Slowly, but surely, science is bearing this out.

In this book I try to put together all the facts that I have learned throughout my practice, and my study and research of the past 40 years. I include my own reasoned concepts, as well as the concepts of those brilliant people from whom I have had the good fortune to know.

When speaking about health, we live at a very interesting time.

To put it bluntly, never in our entire history has mankind ever been offered the absolute junk that is now being sold as food in our food stores. These "foods", if we indeed can call them that, are making us fat, lazy and short lived.

In almost all of the industrialized countries, we in this generation are faced with unparalleled decisions concerning our daily food.

Never before has any civilization been exposed to the type of ersatz "foods" and "junk" foods and "dangerous" foods that we are offered. The chips, the sodas, the foods tainted with pesticides, hormones, antibiotics, synthetic colors and flavors. I'm sure you know what I mean.

But conversely never before has any civilization had the opportunity to have some of the best food that ever has been produced, and have it year round. By that I mean we have at our disposal such things as organically grown fresh fruits and vegetables throughout the year, not just seasonal any more. Exotic foods grown or produced in other lands and climates. 'Super phyto-nutrients' and natural food supplements.

From the worst to the best is offered to almost everyone. Our "dilemma" lies in the fact that most people just don't know which is which, nor, how to choose.

It is the object of this book to help you do just that. To help you to distinguish between those items that will make you fat and sickly and short-circuit your life, and those that will create a powerhouse of health and allow you to live a long healthy, vibrant life. To do this you must start making the right decisions with everything that goes into your mouth.

Unfortunately, much of the advertising we are exposed to on a daily basis can be misleading if not downright false. You must learn to be discriminating! What's more, your life and health depend on it!

The fact is that you must know enough to be able to make the right decisions, because ultimately when you shop *"the decision is yours"*.

The first rule that I offer is this: Never go shopping at mealtime or when you are hungry.

Secondly don't waste your money or health on negative foods. And third, keep those foods out of your home especially if you have children. Neither you nor they need the extra temptation to munch on the "junkies" between meals or while watching TV.

I challenge you to become aware of what you see in the shopping carts of other shoppers at the supermarkets? What are the things that people are spending their hard-earned money on?

I have a way of rating food on its ultimate value to the human body. I rate foods as a "plus" food; a "zero" food; or a "negative" food. It's not really very hard to do this. Simply try to determine if a food has any intrinsic, nutritional value.

Take for instance vegetables, in my opinion they would be rated obviously as a "plus" food. The same with fish, eggs, poultry, meat, fruit etc. How about potato chips, candy, soda pop, French-fries? I would rate them as "negative" foods since they obviously do more harm than good in the human body.

O.K. how about something like ice cream or frozen yogurt. It is apparent that there is some value in these foods i.e. the calcium and phosphorus and some protein, but the bad seems to out- balance out the good i.e. the sugar and synthetic flavors and colors. So, I write them off as neither good nor bad, but reasonably tolerable by the body so long as they are not overdone.

We have a lot to discuss about food, and this is only a start. We'll soon get into more details.

One more thing before we get started. I have been in this field for many years and critics have chided this type of thinking as "food faddism". My answer has always been this:

Humans have been on this planet for thousands of years living on whole natural foods. Although their diets have typically been far from balanced, they have survived on natural, but limited whole foods throughout that entire time. It has been only within the past 50 to 75 years that we have slipped into the culture of refined, manufactured and adulterated foods.

The dictionary definition for "fad" is "a passing fashion".

When examining the different diets throughout the millennia, I don't think it is stretching it too far to understand which diets and which foods are the fads.

What I would like to do with this book is to share with you my experiences of 40 years of practice. Actually, my professional life was as a chiropractor, though I have done considerable work in "investigative reporting" on my many regular radio broadcasts throughout the years. During this time I have been able to garner a great deal of information about my other loves, clinical nutrition, health and exercise.

From reading my curriculum vitae, you will note that my experience has been rather equal in each of these areas of expertise.

My two daughters, my wife, as well as many of my patients and students have been after me for many years to put this information into book form so that it can be shared with others.

Bear with me with some things. Some of my references have been lost in these past 40 years, however, I will try to authenticate as best I can most of the data. Thanks to the wonderful world of the Internet I have been able to restore most of those records plus many more. When I believe something but rely on my own memory, or if a concept is of my own conjecture, I will state that as well.

At the beginning of each chapter I offer an *"Abstract"*. In essence it is a brief summary of the contents of the chapter. If you like, you may read the abstract to determine if that chapter material interests you, and if indeed you want to delve into the full chapter.

I do believe that you will find answers within these pages that you will not find within any other single book. Apply any or all of these data and ideas. I feel certain that applying some or all of it will to that degree enhance your health and longevity.

2.

Basic Concepts

Abstract

*E*very author and perhaps every person will function under his or her own preconceived or learned concepts. So too, I present you with the concepts of health and nutrition that I have learned and that I function under. You may or may not agree with all of them, but I challenge you to at least consider them. More than 40 years of my life have been devoted to health. During that time I have studied, investigated, and yes practiced on hundreds of thousands of patients and have found these concepts to be valid. Hence, I offer them to you in hopes that they might be useful in your quest for good health.

There are so many food concepts around these days that it is rather hard to keep up with all of them. When we decide to try to learn something about health and nutrition, we are bombarded with a multitude of different ideas. Should we eat a diet of only fresh fruit or just vegetables? Should we stay away from meat? Should we exclude animal products totally? Should we cut out our fats? Should we eat a high carbohydrate diet, a low carbohydrate diet, a diet high in protein? Should we determine what to eat by blood types?

Roger J. Williams well known biochemist in his book "Biochemical Individuality" presents many scientific arguments toward the premise that we are all different biochemically, and I believe strongly that he is right. He states in his book that "all geneticists are agreed that what is inherited by organisms from their forebears is a range of capacities to respond to a range of environments. The characteristics that an organism possesses are fundamentally the outcome of the interaction of heredity and environment." 1

Without a doubt, our familial history over many generations plays a significant role in how our bodies can survive on the food available in the specific geographical area we now live . In other words, where did our parents and grandparents come from? Were they exposed to only very limited specific foods available in that specific local? Their adaptation to certain climates and the conditions and foods available to them in a location is called "*Natural Selection*" By this concept, only those individuals that can survive in that specific geographical area will survive and reproduce other surviving progeny.

If I may, let me give you some basic ideas that might make some sense to you.

Let's start with a very large table filled with only the best organically grown natural foods. No junk here at all. The table is brimming with the best of all types of natural foods from all over the world. You are invited to partake of anything you would like. What would you eat, what *should* you eat?

I like to use my wife and myself in this example.

Sonia comes from Scandinavian stock, only one generation removed. Her Norwegian family we learned, comes from a tiny fjord on the West Coast of Norway called Rekefjord. As far as we can determine her family has lived there for, who knows, perhaps hundreds of generations. The fjord offers some very special characteristics and challenges. The winters are very cold and very long. Conversely, the summers are very short, offering a very short growing season. The one staple that is always available is fish and other products from the sea. Rekefjord actually means "shrimp fjord" so, obviously, shrimp and fish were a large part of their diet in both winter and summer.

We can assume also that vegetables were available, but only for short periods of time in the summer and fall except perhaps for potatoes, turnips and other root crops and berries.

However, these would not be able to be stored and hence would not be available much longer than to mid December. This would mean that from January through April or even May or June, fresh vegetables would simply not be available. Obviously there were no supermarkets throughout those generations, and each family had only that which was grown and stored by them. We sometimes fail to realize that in obscure isolated areas of the world, most families had to be self-sufficient. So let's go back fifteen, twenty, thirty generations. A child is born in that fjord. It must be able to survive in that climate and on the foods available in that fjord. If, for example, that child did not have an immune system that can function with little or no vitamin C for 5 months, it more than likely succumbed to pneumonia, diphtheria, or a host of other immune deficiency diseases. Even deficiency diseases like beri beri from a lack of vitamin B, and scurvy from a lack of vitamin C would present a challenge to survival. So if that child dies, it will not reproduce. Hence, the only people that do survive are those who are specifically adapted by "natural selection" to those conditions in that fjord. If they could not survive, they died. If they were able to, they lived and reproduced.

Carry this now to the present. The only people that survived in that fjord were those who were perfectly adapted to it through natural selection. My wife being one of them. She is the very top of that survival pyramid, adapted to live in that fjord, but here she is now in America, in an entirely different set of circumstances and conditions. So what should she be eating here and now?

In contrast, my family comes from Sicily, a sub-tropical area with the only similarity being the availability of fish, since fish had to be a major part of my family's diet also. Obviously, fresh vegetables and fruits of all kinds were available year-round, including olive oil, tomatoes, figs, nuts, etc.

All right, we've set the stage. We are both standing at the table loaded with the best organically grown foods available. Should she eat the same foods that I eat? Would her body thrive on the same foods that mine will? Does she have the same digestive and absorptive traits as I do?

My common sense answer is obviously NO! We are both survivors, but adapted to entirely different geographical areas of the world, as you are also. Our families have survived for hundreds of years on the foods available where they came from. It makes much more sense to me that this should be our guiding factor when selecting foods that we individually will thrive on. Notice, I'm not saying "survive on" I'm saying "thrive on"

I give you this as only a basic guide, since especially here and now very few people can isolate their backgrounds so purely.

Next, we have to take into consideration our children who are now a mixture of both parents. What should they eat? Which foods will be the best for them? What foods will be best for you? My advice is to get some basic ideas from your heritage, your background, where your families came from. Use that as a guide. Then analyze. Are you a combination of German, English and Irish? Moroccan and French? Try to get some concept of what your family diets must have been. Use that as a starting point. Here's a little tip; if you exercise, especially aerobic exercise, be very conscious of your energy and feelings as you exercise. My sport for many years was swimming laps. On some days after the third or fourth lap, I would feel like quitting, hardly able to continue. Other days, you simply couldn't stop me I felt so good. I have always tried to correlate these feelings with the food that I ate at my previous meals. In other words, certain foods seemed to give me better energy and endurance than others. I suggest that you too become extra aware of your feelings. Even if you are not an aerobic exerciser. Some days you are bound to feel better than other days. Make mental or even written notes of the foods that affect you both good and bad. Test them several times to make sure that your results are consistent. Learn what foods your own body thrives on.

Another way to ascertain the foods that <u>don't</u> agree with you is to try the "Coca Method". With this method, you must first become familiar with your pulse. I suggest your thumb on your wrist (since you will get a double pulse). Take it for one minute or thirty seconds. Once you are able to easily take your own pulse, take it at various times during the day. While sedentary, during light exercise like walking and if you wake up during the night. Almost any food will cause your heart to beat somewhat faster. But if a food causes your heart to beat more than 10 – 15 beats per minute faster than normal during a sedentary time, you are reacting poorly to that food and it probably should be omitted from your diet.

Finally, another method of helping you to ascertain what food you need would be by "cravings". Ah, but here we can be easily misled. If you have a craving for a hot fudge sunday, you can automatically dismiss that as a false craving. (Need I say more)?

Truly I have known pregnant women to show remarkable abilities to crave foods that would give them nutrients that they need. But again, you must be very careful. If the craving is for anything other than a true natural food, it more than likely is false.

We are now at a very unusual time in human social development regarding food.

In one respect, we as a society are being exposed to the largest and most insidious amount of "junk foods" that has ever been offered to any society before. And so many people have succumbed to these "non-foods". When you read the chapters on "Food Additives" and "Meat" you will get an idea of just what I am talking about. The next time you are shopping at the supermarket, take a quick look at the carts around you. See how so many people are addicted to, and wasting their money on these "non-foods", yes even dangerous foods. On the other hand, looking at the bright side, we as a civilization have available to us a fantastic array of wonderful foods, the breadth of which has never been offered to any society before. Fresh vegetables and fruit, year 'round, no matter where you are in our country. We have available to us nuts, figs, dates, olives, coconuts and so much more from other areas around the world. Furthermore, never has mankind been offered the wide range of phytonutrients that we now have such as carrot juice, CoQ10, grape seed concentrate, odorless garlic, blue green algae, barley grass concentrate and so much more (check the chapters on food supplements and herbs). You have the option to choose the best or the worst, which puts you into a very unique position that no other culture, has ever had before.

As a general rule, always keep this short phrase in mind when shopping "buy foods that are as fresh as possible, with the least amount of adulteration, contamination and additives". Bear in mind another general rule, "your best foods are usually fresh, if however they are not available, then frozen, only then, if not available, canned."

Let's look at my example of apples.

You are walking in your large field in late summer. Ahead of you is that apple tree your grandfather planted many years ago. It's growing on rich deep alluvial soil. The field and tree have never had chemicals used on them. You go over to that tree and see that it is laden with the most delicious apples, and they are all ripe. You reach up and pick one and eat it on the spot. Delicious can't be better. The juices are drooling down you chin. You eat another. You can't do any better than that. Organic apples picked at their peak of ripeness, eaten immediately.

But you liked it so much that you pick more of them, filling all of your large pockets, inside your shirt, and anywhere else you can put them. The day is hot; you walk back to the house about 1/4 mile away. By the time you get to the house, you are sweating and hot. You decide to eat another apple. It tastes wonderful, but if we were able to micro-analyze it for nutritional content, it would have an infinitesimally lesser nutritional value because of the heat from the day and from your body. But that's O.K. because it still has an abundance of nutrients. Now you start thinking about making a delicious apple pie.

Immediately, you start by peeling and coring the apples, as you do, you put the finished pieces on the counter beside you. You then notice that they are beginning to turn brown (oxidation). Nevertheless, you eat a piece. It is still very delicious and nutritious, but not as nutritious as the one you ate when you got home, or the one you ate right off the tree. So you finish the pie and put it into the oven. When it comes out, you must have a piece (as I would).

But, though still rather nutritious, after the cooking, it doesn't have near the nutritional value that the piece on the counter had, nor the one you ate as you got back to the house and certainly not as much as the one you ate off the tree. But, you still have some apples left, so you decide to make some apple sauce. You pare the apples, cut them, cook them, mash them, put them in jars, and boil them in your canning pot. And when finished, you store them down in your cellar. Several months later in the cold of winter, you decide to open one of the jars. Is there any nutritional value in that applesauce? Certainly some, but not nearly as much as in the apple pie, or the one you ate while paring them etc. etc. Think of this story when you are deciding which foods to buy at the supermarket. Every type of processing that a food undergoes takes its toll on the embodied nutrients.

Another bit of help in selecting food would be; Fresh first; frozen next; canned last.

3.

The Immune System

Abstract

W*hether talking about cancer, bacteria or viruses or indeed anything that challenges our lives, the immune system is involved in protecting us.*

In this chapter we discuss many of the factors such as antibiotics drugs, stress and even sugar that compromise or damage this system as well as those factors such as nutrients, fever, fasting and even prayer that strengthen it. The information is vital to everyone who chooses to become and stay healthy. At the end of this chapter we give you an immune enhancing drink that has kept my patients and family away from the overuse of antibiotics.

One system of the body that we should all become familiar with is the immune system.

Simply defined, the immune system is a part of our body that protects us from internal and external factors that would or could harm us. Whether we are referring to environmental pollen and bacteria externally, or cancer cells within us, it is the job of the immune system to help us to survive. There are many factors that enhance the immune system, and many factors that damage or compromise it. The following discussion addresses examples of some of the many factors.

IMMUNE SUPPRESSING FACTORS

A. Antibiotics and some drugs

As we discuss in our chapter on meat, antibiotics have been greatly overused and misused. We can cite many examples to show that although antibiotics have been touted as "miracle drugs," and indeed they are, that when overused they can also do a great deal of harm to the body and to our environment.

(1)   Suppression of the immune system

In many cases, antibiotics actually suppress the production of antibodies. For example, Tetracycline has been shown to inhibit the ability of white cells to engulf and destroy bacteria (called phagocytosis), as well as to delay the ability of white cells to move to the site of an infection.

Some common antibiotics such as the Sulfonamides were found to inhibit the microbiocidal activity of the white cells. This simply means that the white cells that engulfed these bacteria were less able to destroy them. Trimethoprim sulfamethoxazole was found to actually inhibit antibody production. Similar actions were found with numerous other antibiotics. [1]

The use of antibiotics has been shown to increase the likelihood of repeat infections. Children with strep throat who were given antibiotics recovered from the initial infection in short order. However, **they experienced a rate of recurrent infections two to eight times higher than those children not receiving antibiotics at all.** [2]

Even the U.S. Department of Health and Human Services now discourages antibiotics for Otitis Media (ear infections). They state that most cases resolve spontaneously without antibiotics. Because of this, and because of the potential of the development of further microbial resistance to antibiotics, the U.S. Department of Health and Human Services is now discouraging the treatment of ear infections with antibiotics. [3]

In yet another study, **children with chronic earaches who received antibiotics experienced two to six times more recurrent ear effusion than those receiving a placebo (a sugar pill).** 4

One of the apparent puzzles in medicine is the problem that is called Chronic Fatigue Syndrome. As the name implies, the patient with this condition experiences constant overwhelming and continual fatigue. I have had patients who have suffered with this for many years, with some doctors even refusing to admit that their condition was real. In one particular study, 80 percent of patients suffering from Chronic Fatigue Syndrome had a history of recurrent antibiotic treatment. 5

(2)   The proliferation of yeast

Candida is a systemic yeast infection involving the entire body. It is said to cause a variety of symptoms such as gastrointestinal distress, fatigue, lethargy, depression and irritability. It is also suspected to be caused by prolonged antibiotic therapy. This concept was presented by Dr. Leo Galland, M.D., who found that antibiotics were indeed the precipitating factor in 82 percent of Candida-related Complex (CRC.) 6

(3)   Destruction of beneficial bacteria

We all have *e coli* in our intestinal tracts. This is quite normal and expected. We have a variety of other bacteria there also. This too is quite normal. But some years ago, due in part to the indiscriminate use of antibiotics in medicine, but even more so to the agricultural use of antibiotics to increase growth in cattle, a mutant variety of *e coli* has inadvertently developed. This mutant variety is called *e coli* 0157H7. Unlike simple *e coli* and most other organisms, ***e coli* 0157H7 cannot be killed with antibiotics,** and to make matters worse, **it produces a deadly toxin.** Perhaps it would be more precise if the mutant variety had a different name since it is entirely different from simple *e coli*.

All of this seems bad enough, but the plot thickens: a person who becomes infected with *e coli* 0157H7 by eating tainted meat will be compromised, *but the greatest danger is to take oral antibiotics.*

This would be the scenario:
The person eats the infected meat, allowing 0157H7 entry into the intestine. A small quantity producing some toxin can make the person mildly to moderately sick, depending on how much is present. But the 0157H7 bacteria are competing with and being held in check by all of the other good bacteria present; especially those producing lactic acid like yogurt.

If then, for perhaps another illness, his physician gives this person some oral antibiotics, the result would be that the antibiotics would kill off all of the other good bacteria in the intestine, all except 0157H7, since, being resistant to antibiotics, it would be unaffected. Without any competition, the 0157H7 variety multiplies exponentially, creating a great deal of toxin; either killing or making the host terribly sick. (For further explanation see our chapter on meat.)

In my opinion, anyone infected with or even suspected to be infected with this organism should take an abundance of probiotics such as yogurt, acidophilus or kefir. These beneficial organisms will offer competition and keep 0157H7 in check.

(4) The promotion of antibiotic resistant bacteria

In an article from the *New England Journal of Medicine*, we are told that the process of "genetic transfer" is rather widespread in nature. Because of this phenomenon, the property of antibiotic resistance can be transferred from one species of bacteria to another, so that the continued use of antibiotics tends to favor the emergence of an array of resistant species 8. In other words, the more we use and abuse antibiotics, the more resistant varieties of microorganisms will be created. It is imperative that the abuse of antibiotics be curtailed.

B. The effects of sugar

One of the most profound studies that I have yet come across involves our body's ability to fight off infection by what is called "phagocytosis." Phagocytosis is the ability of certain white blood cells to surround, engulf and destroy bacteria and other foreign bodies in our blood. A phagocytic index has been developed which measures this "search and destroy" capability by microscopically visualizing these special cells. By counting the number of foreign bodies within these phagocytes, an index of 15.5 was found to be normal in most human beings. However, in a study done by A. Sanchez and colleagues, that index was found to drop to about 8.6 with a 100-milligram intake of table sugar (about eight tablespoons). The precipitous drop in the index occurred within one hour, and the normal immunity did not return fully for another five hours! 9

What this means essentially is that when you eat *any* amount of sugar, you compromise your immune system to a lesser or greater degree depending on the amount consumed. As an example, check with friends and relatives to see when their children become sick. More than likely, there was an excessive exposure to sugar. The most obvious times that children get sick are around Easter and Halloween when children are known to consume the greatest amounts of sugar.

Of still greater importance and tragedy is the situation with infant formulas. Read the labels, and you will find that sugar is one of the top two ingredients. Remember that the effects of a dose of sugar on the immune system last for up to five hours. If an infant is on a 2-3 or even 4-hour feeding schedule, the child may never be at its full immune potential. Considering these facts, is it any wonder that the incidence of ear infection in children is so great?

Let's consider the health of older children, using soda pop alone as an example. First of all is the fact that in the year 2000, the consumption of soda pop accounted for more than a quarter of all beverages consumed in the United States. More than 15 billion gallons were sold in that year alone. Statistically, a full third of all teenagers in the U.S. drink at least three cans of soda pop each day. In order to give you some concept of just how much sugar that is, consider that one 12-ounce can of soda pop contains 10 teaspoons of sugar. Therefore the average teenager is getting about 30 teaspoons of sugar from his or her three cans of soda. 10, 11

Now I'll just mention another substantial health problem. Each 12-ounce can of cola contains, in addition to the sugar, 35-38 milligrams of caffeine, which is a little more than a quarter the amount found in a typical cup of coffee. Most parents will restrict the consumption of coffee with their children, but have no restrictions whatsoever when it comes to soda pop and colas. Caffeine stimulates the secretion of stored sugar from the liver into the blood, which adds further to the immune challenge. The introduction to caffeine in children also sets the stage for the dependence on caffeine in later years.
(See our chapter on emotional illness.)

C. <u>Nutritional Deficiencies</u>

There are many specific nutrients that play a part in supporting the immune system.

As has been suggested by many studies, the leading cause of immune breakdown is poor nutrition. Vitamin, mineral and protein deficiencies are major factors in compromising the immune system. This is discussed more completely below in the section on nutrients that enhance optimum immune function.

12

Other nutritional immune suppressors that I have come across in my studies are the following: excess polyunsaturated fats (oils such as peanut, sunflower and safflower) as well as the minerals nickel, excess zinc, cadmium, mercury, arsenic, and excess copper.

D. Stress

Stress in human terms is when a person is subjected to disquieting or disruptive influences. These can be mental, emotional, or physical.

The most important pioneer in understanding the influence of stress on the human body is a researcher by the name of Hans Selye, M.D. simply stated, he named three stages in the stress reaction. He calls these stages "The General Adaptation Syndrome." The first stage is called the "alarm reaction." This is a set of reactions that combat the stress. During this stage, the immune system usually becomes depressed, making us more susceptible to infection and disease. If the stress is not long lasting, we usually recover rapidly. In the second stage called the "resistance phase" when stress lasts longer, our bodies adapt as the immune system works overtime for our "survival". If however, the stress factors are continued willingly or unwillingly for a long period of time, we eventually go into the third stage called "exhaustion." During this stage, our immune system, unable to keep up with the biochemical and neurological demands of the stress, eventually breaks down and begins to fail.

I mention this General Adaptation Syndrome because I believe that there can be a positive effect inherent in the second phase. Fasting (remaining away from all food) can create a beneficial effect by forcing the body into the resistance phase, when the immune system sets itself at high alert for the protection and survival of the individual. A fast lasting of between 36 and 60 hours *does* increase the immune bodies of our defense system. Fasting any longer than 60 hours however, causes the immune system to suffer. 13

Here are some additional references concerning stress and its effects on the immune system that you might find interesting: that psychological stress indeed has a marked effect on immunity 14; that seasonal patterns of stress have an effect on immunity 15 ; and that stress may indeed increase susceptibility to disease. 16

IMMUNE ENHANCING FACTORS

Now that we have given you an idea of the many factors that compromise the immune system, let's discuss the factors that enhance it.

A. The effects of fever

How often have you heard comments by doctors such as "let's get that fever down."?
Or, "take a couple of aspirins to bring the fever down." We are now learning that this might possibly be the exact opposite of what you really should do. Even though there still seems to be some controversy within the medical community, there are many references that indicate the value of fever in enhancing the immune system. Surely, when the fever is brought lower by the action of aspirin and other NSAIDS (non-steroidal anti-inflammatories) the patient *feels* more comfortable. But the general consensus seems to be that when you bring the fever down, you also increase the duration of the infection. 17

There also seems to be some controversy concerning how high a fever should be allowed to go before something is done to bring it down. In my practice throughout the years, I have used the figure of 103°F-104°F as a guiding point at which I will bring the fever down. Also, rather than using an NSAID, I have always used a tepid bath or cool towels to do this. The caution is to prevent the patient from going into chills. If that happens, the patient should be put under warm blankets. It is essential to remember that if a patient is at risk for seizures, one must be very careful about how high the fever should be allowed to go.

Of all of the references that I have seen, the one that presents the information most clearly is the article that appeared in *Science Magazine* by Edwin Kiester, Jr.
I will paraphrase it as follows:

"After the arrival of a foreign substance into the blood stream, a chemical called *endogenous pyrogen* (Greek for 'fire within') is released from white blood cells, and quickly takes command of the body's defense system. It raises the temperature in the hypothalamus by means of activating prostaglandins. As well as causing an elevation in temperature, E.P. itself helps step up the production of T-cells, which are a vital part of the immune system. It has been shown that T-cell production increases 20-fold when the temperature is raised from 98.6°F to 102.2°F. Elevated temperature also strengthens the effect of the antiviral agent *interferon* which is more than three times as effective when the temperature is raised from 102.2°F to 104°F". 22

The point that I am trying to raise here is that for as many years as I can remember, we have been told that we should do everything to get the fever down, when it appears now that this is the exact opposite approach that we should be taking. If you are inclined to understand the exact mechanism as to how this fever is produced in the body, as well as the specific effects that fever has on the immune system, you might take a look at the references cited here.18,19, 20, 21

B. Fasting

We mentioned briefly above that fasting has a profound effect on the immune system. Now let me elaborate. First, we should understand the exact definition of fasting.

Various dictionaries define it differently. Some regard a fast as "the abstaining from certain foods for a period of time." Others refer to a fast as "the total abstinence from all foods but not water." This latter definition is the one that we will proceed under.

Some writers use the terms "fasting" and "starvation" synonymously. There is nothing further from the truth, even though the application is the same. Let me explain by giving you an example. Let's say that we conscript two individuals by offering each a thousand dollars to participate in our experiment. We make it clear to each that there will be no turning back once they have committed. We then take each subject into separate rooms and give the following instructions separately. To the first one we say, "You have voluntarily agreed to do exactly what we want. You will be used in an experiment to see if a person will starve by going 10 days without food. Now we won't let you die, but we will let the experiment go as long as we can. You can however have all the water you want."

To the second person we say, "You have volunteered for this experiment. We want you to fast for 10 days. Fasting can be very healthy for you since you will be cleansing the body, perhaps prolonging your life, and definitely enhancing your immune system. In addition to these benefits, you definitely will experience a loss of weight. These are the stages you will go through, and these are the things you must do, and must not do".

The responses from each of these individuals in the next few days will be will be vastly different. The first individual, having had no previous experience of going without food for longer than overnight, will soon start to have feelings of hunger, which will gradually get worse. As they intensify, he starts 'imaging' food, which causes the problem to further worsen. As he thinks about food, his digestive secretions and contractions increase in anticipation of food. His stomach churns, his mouth salivates. Eventually, not understanding the mechanisms of fasting, he will start to become afraid, and the fear will cause a release of adrenaline. Soon he will go into a full-blown anxiety attack, the results of which could indeed cause death if it were allowed to continue. I have read stories of people who have died of "starvation" after only several days! The truth is that they died of fright and anxiety, not starvation. Although I personally have never fasted longer than 7 days, I have read where people have fasted for much longer than that. I am not in favor of this, but it indeed can be done without starving to death.

Mental preparation for a fast is vitally important. The second person in our hypothetical experiment, given the right advice as to what to expect, and what to do and not do will avoid the anxiety-produced adrenaline, and should fare quite well.

There has always been a great deal of controversy as to just how long a fast should last. As discussed above in the section on stress, we see that during the second stage of stress described by Selye as the resistance phase, the immune system is enhanced. But after a prolonged period of stress, the immune system eventually breaks down.

These are exactly the responses we get during a fast of differing lengths. A short fast of only several hours has minimal effects on a person. He may go into a phase of low blood sugar (hypoglycemia), which can mildly compromise the immune system. But during a fast of between 36 and 60 hours the response by the immune system is profoundly beneficial. Studies indicate that a fast longer than 60 hours begins to severely compromise the immune system just like any other stress factor would in the exhaustion phase of stress. In other words, fasting acts on the body as a stress factor, having the same effects as any other stress factor, that being the survival of the individual. It seems quite apparent to me that fasting can be used to great advantage as an immune system enhancer if the fast remains within the time parameters of 36 to 60 hours. 23

In a study done at the University of Pittsburgh School of Medicine with 15 human subjects, and with a fast lasting for 14 days, it was shown that immune parameters were improved, with some increasing as much as 24 percent. 24 The study mentions that these results were not consistent. I believe that if the fasting period had ended within the 60-hour parameter, the results would have been considerably better.

It has been shown in many studies that simply restricting calories causes beneficial effects. It was previously thought that the restriction of calories alone was the prime factor in achieving enhanced immune function and longer life. However, it has more recently been shown that there is a marked difference between a simple restriction of calories and in fasting. 23

With a continuous restriction of calories, a person is likely to lose a great deal of weight which could, in the long run go beyond the bounds of sensible moderation, extending into Selye's "exhaustion phase." Whereas in fasting, a person will eventually make up those lost calories at the end of the fast. The most exciting result of a moderate fast is prolonged life. After reviewing many studies involving fasting which yield contradictory results, I maintain that that these differing results are parallel to the reactions that we find in Selye's description of the three stages of stress. 25, 26, 27 So, to sum up let me say that fasting can be a great help in increasing the potential of the immune system. But the ideal duration of a fast must remain within the parameters of approximately 36 to 60 hours, as described by Dr. Selye as the "resistance phase."

C. Nutrients involved with immunity

The importance of a continually strong and properly functioning immune system is closely bound to life itself. The concept that we die of "old age" is very misleading. By that I mean that people mostly succumb to one illness or another. The 96-year-old woman who eventually dies of pneumonia does so because her immune system has more than likely collapsed. The older person who dies of cancer or heart disease does so because the immune system has failed.

I am reminded of a story told by a professor. "There once was a master craftsman years ago who decided to build the perfect (horse drawn) wagon. He selected the finest hard wood, preserving it in special solutions. He used the finest metal available for the wheel rims and hardware. He took the utmost care in the measuring and cutting of each piece fitting everything together perfectly. When it was completed, it was the finest wagon around, and when he died it still was in perfect condition. His son was bequeathed the wagon and he used it for his entire lifetime, and he gave it to his son, and then his son. Thus, it lasted for many generations, functioning perfectly. In the fourth generation thereafter, as the great grandson was driving down the road one day, the entire wagon wood, metal and fittings all turned to dust at exactly the same time".

To explain this metaphor, let me just say that our bodies can be likened to that wagon. Assuming that we are born "perfect", and assuming that we had taken perfect nutritional care of our bodies, then all of our organs should last about the same time. We could then say that we indeed did die of "old age". If you are a Bible believer, then you must take seriously *Genesis 6:3*. The Lord said *"My spirit shall not abide in man forever for he is flesh, but his days shall number 120 years."*

I take this verse quite seriously, and believe that with proper care and nutrition, we each can live that long. And I don't mean in a decrepit way, but functioning rather well for the entire lifetime. To do this however means to consistently maintain a properly functioning immune system. Specific nutrients in proper balance and regular short periods of fasting must be an integral part of our regimen. In a statement made to UNESCO in 1971 by Dr. Alex Comfort of London University College's research group on aging, he confirmed this concept.

He cited "...by the selective use of starvation (fasting) scientists have succeeded in increasing the life expectancy of laboratory animals by as much as 50 percent with a regimen of optimal nutrition and fasting throughout an entire lifetime". If you extrapolate these data, an increase of our general life span by 45-50 percent puts us very closely to the suggested goal of 120 years!

The scientific studies confirming the importance and value of various nutrients in strengthening the immune system are voluminous. I have been collecting these data throughout the years, and list here a few of the pertinent studies that convey the importance of nutrition in supporting the immune system.

Vitamin A
Causes a greater immune response with increased T-cell activity. 28 Vitamin A supplementation reduced the mortality rates from measles by 50 percent. 29 Study results indicate vitamin A treatment might be an important consideration in restoring the depressed immune competence seen in systemic lupus erythematosis. 30

A marginal vitamin A deficiency in children results in compromised immune function. 31

Vitamin B
The results of this study show that improved vitamin B6 status might slow or halt the progressive decline in immunocompetence and improve resistance to colds, infection, and disease in elderly populations." 32

Results of this study indicate that B vitamin supplementation can prevent immune suppression induced by stress. 33

Vitamin C
Because histamine suppresses the activity of the accumulated immune cells, the results of this study support previous findings and show that vitamin C might indirectly enhance neutrophil chemotaxis and enhance the immune response by detoxifying histamine. 34

Vitamin E

These results support previous findings that vitamin E enhances several aspects of immune function, including a stimulating effect on splenic lynmphocytes and alveolar macrophages in the lungs. 35

Beta Carotene

Results here support the hypothesis that the immune system is influenced by beta-carotene, and an optimal dietary intake of beta-carotene might improve immune function. 36

Selenium (a mineral)

The effects of selenium deficiency are far reaching and can involve the heart and muscles by way of free radical and oxidative damage. 37

As a review, let me give you a comprehensive list of all of the factors that are known to affect the immune system.

Enhancers:

Vitamins A; C; E; B6; pantothenic acid; and folic acid

The minerals: selenium; zinc; copper; iron; iodine; magnesium; cobalt Other factors: fasting (36-60 hours); Omega III fish oils; olive oil; glutamine; fever; canthaxanthin (a carotenoid); Coenzyme Q10.

Suppressors:

nickel; zinc; cadmium; mercury; arsenic; sugar; excess copper; stress; excess of polyunsaturated oils.

There are 105,000 references listed in the Google search engine for nutritional influences on the immune system, should you be interested in further research. 38

D. The Effects of Prayer

Some of the most intriguing studies are those that confirm the power of prayer in improving the immune response in patients. Although this perhaps sounds far-fetched, let me give you some details.

A cardiologist by the name of Randy Byrd, M.D., conducted a stringent scientific study involving 393 coronary care patients. Anonymous participants prayed for 192 of these patients each day. Prayers were specific, including the name of the patient, their condition, and a request for beneficial healing and quick recovery. The remaining 201 patients received no prayer. This was a double blind study where neither the doctors involved nor the patients knew which group they were in. The patients themselves were unaware which ones were being prayed for. The test was conducted for ten months. 39

The subjects receiving prayer had significantly fewer complications than the control group and were five times less likely to require antibiotics than those not receiving prayer.

At the present time, there are many more studies confirming and duplicating the work of Dr. Byrd, most of them double blind studies done with humans. 40, 41, 42, 43 This work is so fascinating and compelling that the *Readers Digest* carried a headline article about it in the May 2001 issue. 44

Still skeptical? Why not try it!

Some miracle foods

The next story is strictly anecdotal, and although I have no formal studies, reams of personal cases with family, friends and patients confirm my findings. I have found several foods that so enhance the immune system that the only word to describe them would be miraculous!

When I was finishing my professional training in New York in 1961, my wife gave birth to our second child. At that time there was only one hospital in New York that was delivering "naturally." The unfortunate happened, and she developed a severe breast infection of what is commonly known as "hospital staphylococcus" (a highly resistant variety of staphylococcus aureus.) At that time and still today this is a dreaded infection for anyone in a hospital because it is extremely antibiotic resistant. 45 Nevertheless, a strong antibiotic was recommended for both mother and child.

On the basis of the side effects of such strong antibiotics, I refused treatments and decided to take my wife and new daughter home. At that time my wife was burning up with a fever of 104.5°F. Her breasts were red and swollen and she was unable to nurse. Now that I had her home with me, the next question was "what to do?" I called a professor with whom I had a friendly relationship and he advised me give her several thousand milligrams of vitamin C each hour. As I headed out the door to buy some high potency vitamin C, I had what only can be described as a "divine inspiration."

Something came to me about the white rind of lemons. I headed out the door straight for the pharmacy for some synthetic vitamin C (to the best of my knowledge there is no source of natural vitamin C), then to the fruit stand where I bought a dozen lemons. At home I peeled and discarded the outer yellow off the lemon, leaving as much of the white rind as possible, which I diced and put it in the blender with some water. After blending it to a fine consistency, I gave it to my wife with 2000 milligrams of vitamin C. She drank it with no hesitation. This was at 5:00 pm, and her temperature, as I said, was 104.5°F. Within one hour her temperature began dropping. By 10 pm it had dropped to 100.5°F. I had her sleep through the night with no interruptions. The next morning upon arising, her fever was down to 99.5°F. With some moist heat on her now slightly mottled breasts, she began nursing our infant. We continued the "lemon drink" with vitamin C every three hours that day, and the next day there was no sign of any infection at all! The following day, we received a call from the hospital asking how she was doing. (I'm sure they were expecting the worst.) When I said that she was just fine, with no trace of infection, and that the baby was nursing normally, they asked if she would come back to the hospital for a follow-up examination. She agreed, and upon examination, the consensus was that they must have misdiagnosed the initial condition. *They did not ask her what if anything she had done!*

Since then we have refined the formula, which I give below. For almost 40 years in my practice I have utilized this remarkable lemon drink with the most astounding results. My only comment is, "Just try it!"

Our second story goes thus:
Several years ago, my wife visited her family in the Åland Islands of Finland. I must add here that my wife really enjoys talking. However, one morning while there she awoke with a case of laryngitis, and was unable to speak at all. A true crisis! There in Åland, oranges were not available at the time, so the populace was inclined to drink blueberry juice instead which they have in abundance. Her cousin suggested that she drink several glasses of this and within one hour, her voice had returned. When she returned home several weeks later, she told me the story and I immediately began testing this with our family and suggesting it to patients. Once again, the results were outstanding. Again the best that I can give you is anecdotal evidence, but I certainly invite you to try it. Since then I have been reading other studies that indicate that blueberries contain some remarkable substances, probably flavonoids and bioflavonoids, but we have yet to learn all there is to know about these remarkable berries.

Putting it all together

In refining these two procedures, we have found that a person need only take a third of a blended lemon rind, minus the yellow, (as a matter of taste, the juice need not be included) every three hours with about 1000 milligrams of vitamin C in order to achieve results. Or 1/2 cup of either chewed or blended, frozen or fresh blueberries with 1000 milligrams of vitamin C every three hours. We have found that the blueberries alone will work in most cases, and I suggest the use of blueberries first. Only then, if we are not responding properly do we resort to the lemon rind drink. It is important that these be given with the vitamin C every 3 hours!

Here is a formula for the ultimate best of both:

Lemon /blueberry drink

<u>**Ingredients:**</u>

one thick rinded lemon
1 cup blueberries (frozen or fresh)
Frozen Welch's purple grape juice concentrate (no sugar)
two cups water

<u>**Preparation:**</u>

Peel off the outer yellow from lemon and discard. Leave as much of the white rind as possible. Slice lemon into smaller pieces and put into a blender, seeds, rind and all.

Put blueberries into blender.

Put approximately one inch (from the can) of the frozen grape juice concentrate into blender.

Add two cups of water.

Blend thoroughly.

This makes approximately 4-5 adult doses.

This recipe can be doubled if you have a powerful blender.

Each dose should be taken with vitamin C as prescribed.

Good luck!

Copyright 2003 Dr. Francis J. Trapani

REFERENCES – The Immune System

1. Hauser, W.E.; Remington, J.S., Effects of Antibiotics on the Immune Response. Am. J. Med.; 1982; 72 (S). 711 – 715.
2. Pichichero, M ; Disney, F.A.; Talpey, W.D. et al. Ped. Infect. Dis. J. 1987; 6:635 – 643.
3. Otitis Media with Effusion in Young Children. Clinical Practice Guideline #2. U.S. Department of Health & Human Services. Public Health Service.
4. Cantedin, E.I.; McGuire, T.W..; Griffith, T.L.; Antimicrobial Therapy for Otitis Media with effusion. J.A.M.A. 1991; 266 (23); 3309 – 3317.
5. Case Studies Carol Jessup M.D. Ass't Clin Prof. Univ. Ca. S.F.
6. Leo Galland M.D. Keynote Speaker C.R.C. Convention/ 1988.
7. http://www.ems.org/antibiotics/antibiotics_food.html
8. S.B. Levy N.E.J.M. Sept 6, 1984. 311: 663 664..
9. Sanchez, A., et al Role of Sugars in Human Neutrophilic Phagocytosis Am J. Clin. Nutr.. 26: 1180 – 1184, 1963.
10. http://www.publichealthadvocacy.org/resources/ Soda%20Fact%20Sheet.pdf
11. http://www.cspinet.org/sodapop/liquid_candy.htm
12. http://www.healthy.net/asp/templates/column.asp?PageType =column&ID=64
13. http://www.healthnewsnet.com/gap.html
14. http://www.positivehealth.com/permit/Updates/rudimune. htm
15. http://assets.cambridge.org/052159068X/sample/ 052159068XWS.pdf

16. http://www.acs.ohio-state.edu/units/research/archive/
stressinf.htm
17. http://www.biol.sc.edu/courses/bio102/f97-39.html
18. http://www.merck.com/pubs/mmanual/section13/
chapter150/150d.htm
19. http://jan.ucc.nau.edu/~fpm/bio205/lect25.html
20. http://www.link.med.ed.ac.uk/RIDU/section1.PDF
21. http://www.md.huji.ac.il/microbiology/book/cho49.htm
22. Edwin Kiester Jr. "A Little Fever Is Good For You" Science,;
November, 1984.
23. Sanchez. Et al "Role of Sugars in human Neutrophilic
Phagocytosis" Am. J. Cl. Nut. 26. Nov. 1973. pp. 1180 – 1184.
24. Wing; Stanko; Winkelstein; and Adibi. "Fasting Enhanced
Immune Effector Mechanisms in Obese Subjects". Am. J. of
Medicine Vol. 75.July, 1983.
25. http://www.pnas.org/cgi/content/full/100/10/
6216?ijkey=9868dd902f1ba67816d31037ac577c923e7295b5
26. http://www.healthy.net/asp/templates/news.asp?Id=6609
27. http://www.stopgettingsick.com/templates/news_template.
cfm/6645
28. Nuwayri – Salti N; Murad T. "Immunologic and
Antiimmunosuppresive Effects of Vitamin A.; Pharmacol 1985;
30: 181-187.
29. Barclay A. et al. "Vitamin A Supplements and Mortality
Related to Measles. A Randomized Clinical Trial"; Br Med
J.1987; 294 – 296.
30. Vien C, Gonzales-Cabello R. Bodoi I. Et. al. " Effect of
Vitamin A Treatment on the Immune Reactivity of Patients
with Systemic Lupus Erythematosis" J. Clin. Lab; 1988: 26: 33
– 35.
31. Semba R., Muhilal , Scott A. et. al. "Depressed Immune
Response to Tetanus in Children with Vitamin A Deficiency".; J
Nut. 1992; 122: 101-107.
32. Talbott, M. Miller, L. Kerkvliet, N.; "Pyridoxine
Supplementation: Effect on Lymphocyte Responses in Elderly
Persons". Am. J Clin.N. 1987: 46: 659-664.
33. Lettko, M. Meuer, S. "Vitamin B induced prevention of

stress related immunosuppression: Results of a Double Blind Clinical Study." Ann. N.Y. Acad. Sci. 1990; 585: 513-515.

34. Johnston, C. Martin, L. Cai, x. "Antihistamine Effect of Supplemental Ascorbic Acid and Neutrophil Chemotaxis" J Am Col Nutr. 1992; 11: 172-176.

35. Moriguchi, S,; Kobayashi,N; Kishino, Y: "High dietary Intake of Vitamin E and Cellular Immune Functions in Rats. J. Nut. 1990; 120: 1096-1102.

36. Brevard, P; "Beta Carotene Affects White Blood Cells in Human Peripheral Blood. Nut. Rep. Int. 1989; 40: 139-150.

37. Schrauzer, G.; "Selenium and the Immune Response"; The Health Report; Vol 10 #3.Mar. 1992. (Health Media of America).

38. http://search.netscape.com/nscp_results.adp?source=NSCP Top&query=Immune%20system%20nutritional%20factors&x =12&y=8

39. http://www.webspawner.com/users/apologete2/prayer3.html

40. http://www.ncbi.nlm.nih.gov/entrez/query.fcgi?db=PubMe d&cmd=Retrieve&list_uids=88277956&dopt=Citation

41. http://www.ustoo.com/articles/6c.html

42. http://www.aafp.org/afp/20000201/tips/13.html

43. http://www.salon.com/health/feature/1999/11/03/prayer/print.html

44. Lydia Strohl.; "Why Doctors Now Believe Faith Heals" Readers Digest; May 2001. Pp109-115.

45. http://www.pubmedcentral.nih.gov/articlerender.fcgi?artid=120551

4.

Vitamins, Minerals, and Food Supplements

Abstract

*A*lmost everyone has heard the term "vitamin". In this chapter we give you some background into this vitally important subject. Just what is a vitamin? Where do vitamins come from? How are they used in the body? Is there a difference in the vitamins found in food, and those bought in a store?

The subject of minerals is no less important. Where do minerals come from? How do we get them in our food intake? What are the best sources of minerals for human nutrition?

We suggest that our readers do not use vitamins that are produced synthetically in a laboratory, but rather to use concentrated natural foods that are rich in a specific nutrient. These are available and are called "Food Supplements"

There are several things that you must understand regarding our discussion of this subject. First of all, I will not be discussing specific requirements for each of the vitamins, minerals or other nutrients to any great detail; that information can be obtained from any good nutritional text. I will give general requirements of nutrients and discuss some of the deficiency diseases, clinical and sub-clinical, as well as other things that I feel will help you to better understand the entire concept of human nutrition.

The discovery of vitamins per se dates back to the end of the 19th century. In 1897, a physician named Eijkman discovered that brown rice polishings cured a common condition of the times known as "beriberi." 1, 2

In 1911, a factor was isolated from rice hull polishings by a man named Funk and named "vitamine" under the assumption that it was a life-giving protein or "vita amine." 3 Shortly thereafter, it was discovered that this "growth factor" was actually two separate factors. As the years have passed, other factors have been isolated within that same "growth factor" until now we have a multitude of "B" vitamins commonly called the B complex. It was not until 1936 that the vitamin B1 was synthesized in the laboratory. 4, 5 It is at this point in the evolution of vitamins where I feel that one of the problems in nutrition began. Let me explain.

All vitamins are "organic molecules." This simply means that they are built as a carbon chain or a carbon ring. The carbon atoms form the skeleton for the building of each vitamin. Some of these chemical compounds are very simple, but some are extremely complex. Before a vitamin is synthesized in the laboratory, its chemical structure must first be ascertained by chemical analysis. Then, the chemist finds another "organic chemical" with a similar skeletal structure, and arranges a series of chemical reactions to convert the starting substrate chemical into the synthetic vitamin. Most of these starting chemicals are petrochemicals (from petroleum), and there is considerable controversy as to whether or not these chemically synthesized vitamins are equal to the natural forms. Are the chemical structures exactly the same? Do they react in the same manner as the natural ones in the body? Will they function properly without the synergists that are found in natural foods? 6, 7, 8, 9, 10, 11

Next, I would like you to understand what the very important word "synergist" means. Simply stated, a synergist is a "helping" factor. Synergism describes factors that work together. 12 In nutrition, there is much synergism that takes place. This occurs among the vitamins themselves, as well as with other food factors, such as bioflavonoids and flavonoids. These synergists typically help the vitamins to be absorbed and utilized in the body.

For example, there is much synergy among the B complex vitamins themselves. Deficiency of one B vitamin might create an imbalance of the entire complex. In the same manner, overdosing of a singular B vitamin might also create an imbalance of the entire complex. There is considerable synergy between vitamin C and the flavonoids and bioflavonoids found in Vitamin C-rich foods, just to name a few. 13

Now with that fundamental understanding, let's do an experiment.

To begin, we eat an orange. In that orange we find vitamin C and many vitamin C synergists such as bioflavonoids, rutin, and hesperidin.

We then take a crate of oranges, squeeze them and save the juice. In a laboratory we take that juice and chemically extract from it the pure crystalline vitamin C. This is pure "natural" vitamin C. But the first thing to notice is that we have left behind all of the synergists that usually are available to us in the pulp and rind. Is it natural vitamin C? Yes, indeed, but without the synergists that are usually found in the orange juice. But I must immediately say that this is not the vitamin C that you buy in the store; it is simply too expensive to produce vitamin C in this manner.

However, those natural crystals of vitamin C were studied in the laboratory, and a procedure was determined wherein another chemical is used as the starting substrate. Various chemical procedures are applied to it and eventually a synthetic vitamin C is produced. This is the typical manner in which synthetic vitamins are produced and these are the typical types of vitamins that are commonly sold as vitamins in all stores, including "Health Food Stores."14 These are the types of vitamins that are said to "enrich" certain foods such as breads and cereals. These are also the type of vitamins that are compounded into "multiple" or "one-a-day" varieties.15, 16, 17

As I mention above, some of the vitamins such as vitamin C have very simple structures, and are relatively easy to synthesize. Others like Vitamin B12 and Riboflavin have much more complex structures, and are more difficult to synthesize. I personally am not convinced that the more complex ones truly retain the exact chemical structure as those found in nature. Yet, whether or not they are identical, there are other factors that tend to make me shy away from the synthetic forms. First, as I said, they will not contain the synergists that are found in the natural foods; and second, they are much less likely to be in the same balance as those found in nature. I should note here that these "natural" balances of nutrients found in nature are those that have sustained the human race for thousands of years. In other words, our bodies, our health, our very existence is related to these natural balances.

An excellent example of our inability to duplicate vitamins synthetically is vitamin E. This vitamin is also a complex of certain distinct factors. That which is commonly called vitamin E is actually d- alpha tocopherol. The chemist is yet unable to synthesize the d-alpha form of this vitamin. The best that they can do is to create a similar form called dl alpha tocopherol. When purchasing vitamin E, you will note that some brands say d-alpha tocopherol and some say dl alpha tocopherol, the latter being the synthetic. 18, 19, 20 Furthermore, where vitamin E is found in nature, it is always found with other factors called "tocopherols." These have been labeled from the Greek alphabet, namely alpha tocopherol beta tocopherol, gamma tocopherol and delta tocopherol. Unless you specifically purchase a natural form of vitamin E, these will not be present. It has recently been suspected that the gamma tocopherol might be equally as important or even more important than the alpha tocopherol itself.

With this basic reasoning, early in my practice I decided that there must be a way to get each vitamin in its natural form. I soon found that the only way to do this is to find a "natural food" that is rich in that specific vitamin. Hence, my recommendations for nutritional needs have always leaned towards what we call natural "food supplements." Let me explain what this means. There are certain natural foods that contain very high concentrations of specific nutrients. For example, the richest source in nature for vitamin A is "fish liver oil." The richest sources for vitamin B are brewer's yeast, liver and rice hull polishings. My thinking is this: why take synthetic vitamins when there are such readily available natural sources for most of the vitamins?

In other words, if possible, and when possible, why not use foods that are rich in a specific nutrient rather than use the synthetic forms? By doing this, we know that the chemical formula is correct, that it is in perfect balance, and that any important synergists will more than likely be present. One more thing before we start. Vitamins are divided into two general groups – water-soluble and fat-soluble. Water-soluble vitamins are soluble in water, and fat-soluble vitamins are soluble in fats and fat solvents.

Vitamin A

First of all, vitamin A is a fat-soluble nutrient. What is the best natural source of vitamin A? It has always been fish liver oil. Because oils have the tendency to oxidize and become rancid, I always recommend oils in capsule form. It is simple enough to purchase fish liver oil capsules of vitamin A in the proper dosages. Because it is obtained from a natural food, we know that the vitamin is "natural" and we can expect that if any synergists are involved, they will also be in that oil. Fish oil therefore can be considered our best vitamin A "supplement.

The synthetic form made in a laboratory is called Vitamin A "Palmitate." There are some studies indicating that indeed, there is a considerable difference between the synthetic and the natural forms. 21

Vitamin B complex

The B complex vitamins are called "water soluble" vitamins because they will dissolve in water.

As I mentioned above, the B vitamins are actually a complex of many factors, such as B1, riboflavin, niacin, B6, and B12.. From the discovery of the "growth factor" in rice bran in 1897 until now, scientists throughout the years have managed to isolate each of these separate B vitamin factors. Each discovery has arisen from one of only a few substrates or foods. These are yeast, liver, rice bran, and wheat germ. In other words, each specific B vitamin was isolated from within one of these natural, whole foods. Furthermore, since there have been many years between the discovery of each of these nutrients, (the most recent B vitamin was isolated only several years ago) there may be many others that have yet to be discovered and isolated, so we are not necessarily complete!.

Suffice to say that if and when other B vitamins are discovered, it stands to reason that they will more than likely be found within these same foods. Taking the premise that I mentioned above, that the B vitamins function synergistically together, it seems obvious that only those that have been discovered or recognized can be synthesized. 22, 23, 24 It further follows that the complex cannot be properly balanced using synthetic forms if indeed there are other factors that remain to be discovered in the future.

My point is this: if indeed all of the B factors known today have been isolated from very specific foods, why bother with the synthetic forms with their potential problems, when you can very easily take one or more of the highly nourishing food supplements from which they are all derived? Hence, my recommendation is to simply use one or more of the foods mentioned above that are very high in B factors. The two that I use and recommend mostly to my patients and students are good quality, true brewer's yeast powder (a byproduct of the brewing industry) and desiccated (dried powdered) liver tablets. I take both, simply to be assured that the balance is perfect.

A note must be made here about brewer's yeast. Originally, the health benefits of brewer's yeast were bestowed on pigs! As I understand it, years ago breweries made real beer in large wooden kegs as a combination of various grains and hops. As the beer fermented producing the "brew," it formed a foam head at the top of the barrel. At various stages, the biermeister would use a wide paddle to swab off this head and drop it next to each barrel where it would dry. As a mound accumulated, rather than throw it away, because it was found to be of great nutritional value for pigs and other animals, it was fed as such. Some brilliant soul apparently realized its nutritional value for humans as well. The only problem with the "true" brewer's yeast is that it is extremely bitter. The good news however is that the bitter fraction can be removed without apparently influencing the nutritional value to any great extent. This true brewer's yeast is now recognized by the word "debittered."

Next, let's go back to wartime Germany. During World War II, in a search for inexpensive sources of protein and vitamins, Hitler instructed some of his scientists to solve this food requirement. The result of this investigation was to use an inexpensive substrate (a starting carbohydrate source) and then to grow the beer yeast (saccharomyces cerevisiae) on it. The concept sounds fascinating, but the substrate used was wood chips or sawdust that was then treated with an acid (hydrochloric or sulfuric) to break down the complex carbohydrates of the wood into simple carbohydrates that the yeast can grow on. This method is now also used with other substrates to produce what is called "primary grown" yeast.

Using the same concept developed by the German scientists, various varieties of yeast other than saccharomyces cerevisiae and different substrates are currently used to grow a better tasting yeast. Some of these substrates are molasses and whey, and yes, still wood chips! Indeed, they have come up with better tasting products, but is there a difference? I believe that there is. If we talk about feeding an animal or even a plant a nourishing diet to produce a better quality end product, wouldn't the same hold true for yeast? In other words, would you expect the same nutritional quality in a yeast product made on and from wood chips as you would from yeast made from a combination of many grains and hops? I wouldn't! The fact is that in my forty years of practice I have found a great difference in these products by the effects they have had on my patients. Hence, when buying a brewer's yeast, be sure that it is a byproduct of the manufacture of beer. It will invariably be labeled "debittered"

Vitamin C
Vitamin C is also a water-soluble nutrient. I mention vitamin C above as being a very simple molecule to reproduce synthetically, and it is. The one problem again is that the pure synthetic vitamin C generally does not contain any of the natural synergists. I utilize this synthetic vitamin C mostly because it is the only type available, and also because I believe that when the required synergists are taken with it, it can still be quite effective. Since there are no available natural "food supplement" sources for vitamin C, I recommend that you purchase a vitamin C that comes with its natural synergists — flavonoids, bioflavonoids, rutin, and hesperidin.

Please see the chapter on "The Immune System" for the most advantageous uses of Vitamin C.

Vitamin D
Like vitamin A, vitamin D is also a fat-soluble nutrient. Also like vitamin A, its best source is fish liver oil. Hence when you

buy your vitamin A fish liver oil, buy the one that also contains vitamin D. See our lists below for our recommendations of amounts to be taken.

Vitamin E
Vitamin E is another fat-soluble vitamin. As mentioned above, vitamin E can be purchased in either the natural form or the synthetic form. Currently, most natural vitamin E in supplements are derived from soybean oil. If it is derived from natural sources, the label will state "d-alpha tocopherol." If it has been manufactured synthetically, the label will state "dl alpha tocopherol." That is your major clue to its source. Secondly, the naturally derived forms will invariably contain the other parts of the natural complex. Those are the other tocopherols — beta, gamma and delta. So, a naturally derived vitamin E will be labeled as "d alpha tocopherol in a base of mixed tocopherols" or "with mixed tocopherols." You will therefore recognize the natural form of vitamin E by the words "d alpha" and "with mixed tocopherols."

Vitamin E, whether natural or synthetic, can come in three forms: tocopherol, tocopheryl acetate, and tocopheryl succinate. The tocopherol and tocopheryl acetate forms are oil. The succinate is a dry powder form that is incorporated in tablets rather than in capsules. In any case, the crux of the matter is found in the "d-alpha" or the "dl alpha" on the label preceding each of the three forms listed above, indicating respectively the natural and the synthetic varieties.

The Minerals
Unlike the vitamins, which are rather complex structures, the minerals are rather straightforward. Minerals are those elements that we find on our planet in rock, in the soil and in the sea. All tissues and internal fluids of our body contain varying quantities of minerals. Minerals are constituents of the bones, teeth, soft tissue, muscle, blood, and nerve cells. They are vital to overall mental and physical well-being. In addition to

utilizing minerals such as calcium, phosphorus and magnesium as building materials for our skeletal structure, we also need trace minerals which act as catalysts for many biological reactions within the body, including muscle responses. These trace minerals are responsible for the transmission of messages through the nervous system, the production of hormones, digestion, and the utilization of nutrients in foods. As with so many things, there are some minerals that do the body harm such as lead and mercury and a number of others. However, for good health, the body must have access to most minerals. There are several keys to making the right choices for our supplemental use. I list the vital trace minerals below.

Minerals are found in many sources in nature. The three most important sources are the soil, groundwater and seawater. All soils on the planet are not the same — some have a wide variety of the trace minerals, while other soils are lacking in certain important trace minerals. But it is not commonly understood that most plants can grow and even thrive in the absence of many of the trace minerals. As an example, hothouse tomatoes will grow and flourish with only specific minerals added to the nutrient water. Most farmers will add only nitrogen, potassium and phosphorus fertilizers to their fields. In the Pacific Northwest, our soils are extremely deficient in the mineral selenium. **If a mineral is not in the soil, it will not be in the plants that grow on that soil.** The same holds true for each of the trace minerals. 25, 26

Rainwater is entirely free of all minerals, yet as rain falls onto the soil and begins to percolate downward, it dissolves minerals in the soil. Hence, groundwater contains a multitude of minerals leached from the soil that it has passed through. These are basically dissolved rock minerals. Although the human body can utilize these dissolved minerals, their absorption is not great.

A much better source of minerals for human nutrition is from plants, provided the plants are grown in a soil containing all of the essential minerals. Minerals that have been absorbed by plants and incorporated in their cellular structure are considerably more easily absorbed by the human digestive system than are the minerals from groundwater. These complex compounds that become part of the plant's structure are referred to as being chelated (KEE-lated). When purchasing a mineral supplement, whether it be to satisfy a singular mineral need, or a multi-mineral need, be sure that the minerals are chelated.

The final destination of all of the rainwater that falls on the continental masses is the ocean. As rainwater ultimately reaches the ocean it carries with it all of the minerals that have leached into it from the soils it has passed through. Hence, **the ocean is the ultimate repository for all the minerals from all of the continental masses on the planet.** Unfortunately for us, because seawater is saline (salty) it cannot be drunk. However, things that grow in the ocean contain the full spectrum of minerals. Fish contain many minerals, but **an even greater source of chelated minerals are the ocean plants. Seaweed!** The ocean water continuously bathes each plant with mineral-rich water. When these plants are harvested and washed, the minerals are available without the salt. In fact, there is a balance of all minerals from all of the continents. A more complete source of chelated minerals you cannot find.

Omega III fatty acids

In my opinion, the discovery of the Omega III fish oils may well be the most important discovery of the past 100 years. That's a pretty strong statement, but what the studies have shown us thus far is absolutely amazing! The only problem is that their extraordinary values are not being fully recognized or utilized by the general public. I have maintained for years that if the true value and importance of the Omega III fatty acids we were extolled and the general public was convinced to use them, we would be able to virtually eliminate most heart disease and stroke. But let me not get ahead of myself. Let's start from the beginning.

For many years it was recorded that the Greenland Eskimo population had the lowest coronary heart disease rate in the world! When this was first recognized, several scientists went to Greenland and learned that about 70 percent of their caloric intake was from fat. They extrapolated that increased fat consumption would be the solution to the coronary heart disease problem. They soon learned otherwise. In other words, increasing the intake of the type of fats that our temperate climate produces only made matters worse. It was not until years later that we came to the recognition that all fat is not the same, and that something in the fat of the Greenland Eskimo diet was different. By studying the biochemistry of this fat, it was determined that it contained some very interesting fatty acids.

In biochemical terms fatty acids are factors that fat is made of. In temperate climates, plants and animals form specific types of fatty acids such as oleic, linoleic linolenic, and arachidonic acids. These are developed principally in response to moderate climate. But, the fatty acids produced in the extreme cold climate of the Arctic, and which are part of the Eskimo diet, are unique. They are called eicosapentaenoic acid and docosahexaenoic acid, abbreviated respectively "EPA" and "DHA". 27, 28, 29

One aspect of the biochemistry of fat is that each type of fat has a different "melting point." This is the temperature at which the liquid fat becomes solid or vice versa. As an example you might recognize that if coconut oil is kept in an air-conditioned room it will solidify. Even olive oil if kept in a refrigerator will get cloudy (the first stages of solidifying). But the Omega III oils will stay liquid at even very cold temperatures. The natural origin of these oils begins in the very cold waters of the Arctic Ocean, within tiny organisms called "plankton." These are then eaten by the "krill" which are then eaten by the herring, and so forth up the food chain through the salmon, the seals and whales. The point is that nature provides a fat for the sea creatures in those frigid arctic waters that will not harden even at extremely low temperatures. It follows of course that many of these sea creatures are eaten by the Eskimo who benefit from these very specific fatty acids.

It must be made clear that the Omega III oil we are talking about is the body oil of the fish, and not the fish liver oil! (Fish liver oil is the major source of natural vitamins A and D.)

Omega III oil has a very interesting effect in the human body. The platelets in our blood normally form clots at the time of an injury in order to prevent blood loss. This is called "platelet aggregation." These platelets release their chemicals upon impact or exposure to air. They get sticky and form clots. The important platelet chemical that causes the blood to clot is called thromboxane, and is formed from the fatty acids of our food. Also, in order to prevent too much clotting, we have a "countering substance" in our blood called "prostacyclin." This helps to prevent unwanted clots within the circulatory system. It is essential that a fine balance of these two chemicals be maintained. 30, 31, 32, 33

The clotting reaction can occur at different times and for different reasons. In addition to being released during an injury, platelets can rupture within the circulatory system by striking various "Y"s in the arterial tree as the vessels get smaller and smaller. When thromboxane is derived from solid fats like lard and beef fat, the resultant thromboxane released is very clot prone, and the countering substance prostacyclin is not able to dissolve the clot thoroughly.

Omega III oils have very special effects on our blood clotting systems. The clotting is less intense, and anticlotting is more exaggerated. Hence, by utilizing the special effects that Omega III oil has on our clotting function, we can prevent the major cause of death in the United States, which originates from platelet aggregation, or blood clots, in our coronary vessels, brains, and lungs. Some human studies have been done which require the subjects to eat more fish. The results were less than exciting. However, as with many studies, the correct parameters were not followed. The key to the prevention of coronary disease is not just "eating fish", but rather eating fish containing the Omega III fatty acids .

One of the major producers of the Omega III oils for human consumption, Seven Seas Health Care, Hull U.K., (distributed by R.P. Scherer, Inc.) harvests their fish only in the winter and early spring when arctic waters are coldest. Obviously, that is the time when the fish have accumulated the greatest concentrations of the Omega III oils. So, while fish is the primary source of these oils, certain fish have greater quantities of body oil than others, and the fish must be harvested at the proper time. Add this effect with the similar effects that vitamin E has on preventing clots, and I believe you can reduce your chances of death from a blood clot in your heart, your lungs or your brain to virtually nil. (See the chapter on Cardiovascular Disease.)

The Carotenoids
Carotenoids are a group of factors found in many foods that when totaled may number well over 700. Of these, 50-60 are present in a good diet containing sufficient fruits and vegetables. There are about 20 carotenoids found in human blood, derived from our diet. They are fat-soluble pigments and are important in human as well as animal health.

When carotenoids are mentioned, we commonly think of beta carotene, but many others are being recognized for their health benefits as well. These are lycopene, canthaxanthin, zeaxanthin, astaxanthin, lutein and beta cryptoxanthin, alpha carotene, delta carotene, gamma carotene, fucoxanthin, capsanthin, crocetin, sulforaphane, bixin, capsorubin, volaxanthin and phytoene.

They are some of our most protective nutrients with health benefits ranging from their ability to reduce the incidence of cancer, to preventing stroke, heart disease, eye disease, and in general enhancing the immune system.

Some of the richest sources of carotenoids are carrots, tomatoes, pumpkin, egg yolks, spinach, sweet potatoes, watermelon and certain fruits such as oranges, mango, papaya, and peaches.

At present, many of the carotenoids are being synthetically produced. There is a strong possibility that some of them might indeed be toxic when taken alone in singular concentrations. I believe that even those carotenoids used as supplements and touted as being from natural sources may offer problems, due to the methods and chemicals used in isolating them. 34, 35, 36, 37, 38, 39

As usual, my recommendation is to use only the natural forms of carotenoids as derived from vegetables and fruits. Of these, carrot juice and tomato juice stand high on my list of "special protective foods."

Once again I reiterate that your best sources for extra or supplemental nutrients are the natural foods and natural food supplements. Indeed, they are more cumbersome to take and there is no way to combine them into one pill. Nevertheless, if you are interested in "the best" then stay with natural foods and natural food supplements for your good health.

General Suggestions for Food Supplements (natural sources for the vitamins)

VITAMIN A	10,000 I.U. capsules fish liver oil	1 daily
CAROTENOIDS	One 6-ounce glass carrot juice	3x per week
VITAMIN B	10 grain Brewers yeast tablets	6 daily
VITAMIN B	10 grain Desiccated liver tablets	6 daily
VITAMIN C	1,000 mg tablets with bioflavonoids	1 daily
VITAMIN D	400 I.U. (in vitamin A capsule)	
VITAMIN E	400 I.U. capsules; d-alpha with mixed tocopherols	1 daily
SELENIUM	200 mcg (chelated)	1 daily
CHROMIUM	100 mcg (chelated)	1 daily
ZINC	50 mg (chelated)	1 daily
MAGNESIUM	500 mg (chelated)	1 daily
CALCIUM	1,000 mg (oyster shell)	1 daily
OMEGA III	1,000 mg (180 EPA; 120 DHA) (capsule)	1 daily
LECITHIN	1,200 mg (capsule)	1 daily
KELP	Tablets*	4 daily
CoQ10	60 mg (capsule or tablet)	1 daily
GINKGO	100 mg (capsule or tablet)	2 daily
SPIRULINA	500 mg	
GRAPESEED (concentrate)	100 mg	1 daily
GARLIC (deodorized)	500 mg (capsule or tablet)	2 daily

These supplements are to be consumed in one day, preferably with food at one or several sittings.

This list is offered to you as a general, non-specific recommendation, for an average healthy adult. But before embarking on any nutritional program, be sure to consult a knowledgeable health minded doctor.

*(Kelp tablets are all of the same size as determined by the maximum amount of iodine allowed in each.)

REFERENCES

VITAMINS MINERALS AND FOOD SUPPLEMENTS

1. http://www.nobel.se/medicine/educational/vitamin_b1/ eijkman.html

2. http://en.wikipedia.org/wiki/Beriberi

3. http://phoenity.com/diseases/beriberi.html

4. Handbook of Vitamins, Minerals and Hormones; R.J. Kutsky; Second Edition.1922; 1973; 1981. Litton Educational Publishing, Inc. p. 216.

5. Nutritional Data; Fourth Edition; Heinz Research Fellowship of Mellon Institute. 1960. P. 30.

6. Today's Dallas Woman, Aug. 1998.

7. http://www.healthbulletin.org/vitamins/vitamins1.htm

8. http://alexia.lis.uiuc.edu/-beiyu/health/ (Natural vitamin E Better retained)

9. American Journal of Clinical Nutrition, March, 1998

10. Dr. Robert Acuff, Ph.D.. Journal of Natural Medicine. November, 1998

11. American Journal of Clinical Nutrition ;1998. Apr,1967;66984

12. http://www.patrickquillin.com/immunopowerchapter_8.htm

13. Handbook of Vitamins, Minerals and Hormones; R.J. Kutsky; Second Edition.1922; 1973; 1981. Litton Educational Publishing, Inc. p. 464.

14. http://www.competition-commission.org.uk/rep_pub/reports/2001/fulltext/456a4.2.pdf

15. http://www.bccresearch.com/editors/RGA-096R.html

16. http://www.sea.siemens.com/chemphar/case/cbchina.html

17. http://www.lhepner.com/food13.html

18. http://www.moormans.com/equine/TechBulletins/VitaminE.htm

19. http://www.getyoure.org/healthpros/back.html

20. http://www.drlam.com/A3R_brief_in_doc_format/2000-No4-VitaminCandE.cfm

21. http://www.megson.com/HYPOTHESIS/MEDICAL_HYPOTHESIS_ARTICLE.html

22. McCormick DB. Riboflavin. in: Shils ME, Young VR. Modern Nutrition in Health and Disease. Lea & Febiger: Philadelphia, 1988, pp. 362-9.

23. Garg R, Malinow R, Pettinger M, et al. Treatment with

niacin increases plasma homocyst(e)ine levels. Circulation 1996;94 (suppl 1):1-457 [abstract #2672].

24. Ubbink JB, Vermaak WJH, van der Merwe A, Becker PJ. Vitamin B-12, vitamin B-6, and folate nutritional status in men with hyperhomocysteinemia. Am J Clin Nutr 1993;57:47-53.

25. http://www.saltinstitute.org/25.html

26. http://lpi.oregonstate.edu/infocenter/minerals.html

27. http://www.ajcn.org/cgi/content/full/74/4/415

28. http://www.ajcn.org/cgi/content/full/ajcn;74/4/464

29. www.issfal.org.uk/Abstracts-Wed.

30. Trapani FJ; Health Discovery of the Century. WCA Journal. 1984

31. Trapani FJ; Eicosapentaenoic Acid and Thromboembolic Disease. ACA Journal; April, 1986.

32. Sanders TAB. Dietary Fat and Platelet Function. Clinical Science(1983) 65, 343 – 350.

33. Eskimo Diets and Diseases. The Lancet. May, 21. 1983.

34. J Nutr. 2004 Jan;134(1):257S-261S.;

35. Int J Cancer. 2004 Oct 28;

36. Int J Vitam Nutr Res. 2004 Mar;74(2):147-52.

37. Br J Nutr. 2004 Jul;92(1):113-8

38. Cancer Metastasis Rev. 2002;21(3-4):257-64.

39. Alves-Rodrigues A, Shao A.,Toxicol Lett. 2004 Apr 15;150(1):57-83.

5

FOOD ADDITIVES

Abstract

In the process of bringing food to your table, many chemicals are used for a variety of reasons. Residual chemicals from the farm such as anti sprouting agents in our potatoes, systemic insecticides and fungicides; coloring agents, flavor enhancers, anti-caking agents, anti-foaming agents, and preservatives. Even packaging chemicals can linger in our food. At one time these were thought to number around 5,000. But now the number is considerably higher. Although we cannot tell you exactly which of these can harm you, you should be aware that these chemicals can have short term and long term reactions as well as interactions. It is not improbable that two or more harmless chemicals can interact to form a deadly one.

As a conservative estimate, there are more than 5,000 chemical substances used in foods in the United States for a variety of reasons. 1, 2, 3 These are governed and controlled by the Food and Drug Administration, which also controls the ingredients in cosmetics. Chemicals are added to preserve the product; to color it, to add to or enhance its flavor; to thicken it, and to prevent caking. Various chemicals are even added in certain bottled products to prevent foaming when it is being put into a bottle. Some of these substances fall into a category called the GRAS chemicals. This means Generally Recognized As Safe. Understand though, they are not *guaranteeing* that they are safe, but only stating that they are "generally recognized as safe". 4 In addition to substances that are added to the food itself, there are also chemicals that the foods come in contact with from packaging, plastics, and machine cleaning agents. 5 The long and the short of it is that there is a long list of chemical additives that end up in the food that we eat.

The question that you may ask about these additives is "so what? Isn't the FDA protecting us? Aren't they all safe?" The answer is definitely NO! 6 Assuming that we eat common store-bought foods, we indeed have the possibility of exposure to many of these chemicals in the course of a typical lifetime.

There are three ways that they might affect us.

Immediate reactions – Let's assume that you ingest a chemical within a particular food that has been incorrectly added. For example, a machine malfunctioned in its preparation and released an inordinate amount of a chemical into a batch of food. That chemical might show no effects in small amounts, but could be toxic beyond a certain limit. When the FDA receives reports of this, they will more than likely have a recall of that batch of food. The FDA has done a good job in protecting us from this sort of mishap.

As an example, while going to professional school, I worked nights at a facility for the temporary detention of juvenile delinquents. Parents would come to visit, laden with all kinds of "goodies." After visiting hour's one day, when all the parents had gone, the kids in my dorm started getting sick and vomiting. Because of the immediacy of the reaction, the sickness could not have been bacterial in origin. Knowing this, I eventually traced the problem to a package of chocolate marshmallow cookies. Every one of the boys who ate any amount of the cookies got sick. This type of case is rather straightforward. However, the next category presents some problems.

<u>Long term reactions</u> – With certain chemicals, reactions might not occur immediately. 7 In other words, it may take repeated doses of the same chemical over a period of time for the cumulative effect to become apparent. Or, perhaps a single dose of a chemical will cause the reaction, but only after it has been in the body for a long period of time. In either case, this type of problem is a difficult one to trace, if indeed it can be traced at all.

Obviously, the FDA is not adept in protecting us from this type of problem. I firmly believe that there are many food additives that fall into categories of being carcinogenic (cancer producing) or causing liver or kidney damage when consumed over long periods of time. Some of these substances have been tested on laboratory animals, but many still remain untested on humans.

A scenario for this type of problem might be, for example, if a person really liked a certain type of food that had as one of its ingredients a specific synthetic color. In small doses, that chemical might be easily tolerated by the body, but repeated doses and its eventual accumulation in the body (lets say in the liver) might result in cancer of the liver in that person.

<u>Interactions</u> – The third problem involving interactions of chemicals should offer us the most concern. In other words, if indeed there are 5,000 chemicals in our foods, and knowing that chemicals have the common habit of interacting one with another, the potential of chemical interactions with 5,000 chemicals reacting with 5,000 chemicals can be staggering!

For example, let's number these chemicals from 1 to 5,000. Chemical 1 can react with chemical 2; number 1 can react with chemical 3; 1 with 4, up to 1 with 5,000. Then 1 and 2 can react with 3; 1 and 2 might react with 4, then with 5, etc. Then 1, 2 and 3 might react with 4, and 5 and 6, etc. The possibilities are astronomical!

The number of potential interactions could be as a mathematician friend of mine speculated "as many as the stars in the sky or grains of sand on the seashore." By his own calculations, this number would be 10^{900} or the digit 1 with 900 zeros after it!

Now, of course, I'm not saying that all of these resultant compounds would be toxic, but surely with that potential number, a good many of them might be! For example when eating a sandwich, what happens if the sodium stearoyl lactylate in the bread combines with the sodium nitrite in the ham, and the calcium disodium EDTA in the mayonnaise? Might there be some interactions? Your guess is as good as mine and equally as good as that of the FDA.

As far as the FDA is concerned, it would be totally impossible to test even a fraction of these, so we are left with no specific protection for interactions. It is interesting to note, however, as I mention in our chapter on meat, that one such inadvertent combination does exist and has been recognized. When the nitrite preservatives in all preserved meat products combine with protein breakdown products called amines in the acid environment of your stomach, deadly systemic carcinogens are formed which are called "nitrosamines."[8, 9, 10] Nitrosamines can cause cancer in any part of the body.

So, what do we do about this problem of food additives? As I have suggested for many years to patients, students, and listeners to my many radio commentaries, "**become label readers.**" Obviously, there is no way that you or I could ever know the exact reactions of each of these chemicals or chemical combinations. So **consider them all undesirable**. Try to use only fresh foods, but if you must buy canned or packaged food, study the label and choose the one with *the least* number of additives.

As an interesting story along these lines, let me tell you about a specific experience we had more than 25 years ago while

I was practicing in Hawaii. It was our family's treat to go out for brunch after church each Sunday. Sonia treated herself to a cup of coffee, but as she was drinking it, she commented that she thought that the cream on the table had gone bad, since the coffee tasted "off." When she commented to the waitress, her reply was that it wasn't cream, but rather the new "cream substitute" which had just hit the market. That incident began my investigation into restaurant additives. Very few people knew then or even know now the extent of chemical ingredients in the foods that we eat in restaurants.

For many years I have taught nutrition classes in the areas where I lived. At that time, and as a result of my radio commentaries, the class I was teaching had several hundred people in it. Of those, over a hundred were students from the University of Hawaii. When speaking about food additives, I happened to mention the cream substitute, as well as other facts that I had learned about restaurant food, including "salad dip" to keep the salad greens crisp without wilting, synthetic bacon chips, the use of monosodium glutamate as a "flavor enhancer" and several others. The class got so upset by this information that they started shouting out "why don't you do something about it, Dr. "T"?

My spontaneous answer was, "Why don't **you** do something about it!" I suggested that we form an investigative committee to analyze the extent of the problem. Immediately, 100+ students volunteered. They agreed to visit each and every restaurant on the Island of Oahu with a survey. It was rather exciting! The students went in pairs to every restaurant on the island. Even though some of the managers were reluctant to give out any information, the results we found were staggering. More than 85% of the restaurants were serving synthetic cream, about the same percent admitted to using monosodium glutamate, about 50% were using salad dip. All of this was done without the knowledge of their patrons. We then managed to get an aggressive state representative on our side who drew up a bill that was then presented to both houses of the state government. It very simply read that all of the items listed on menus in all restaurants throughout the state must list all of the ingredients in each entrée on the menu. You might say that it was the same type of disclosure that we have on canned and packaged foods in our supermarkets.

A hearing was called, at which time we presented our case, and then found that the main opposition to our proposed bill was the Hawaii Department of Health and the local FDA (our protectors). The argument that the opposition presented was that if the bill passed, every large and small restaurant would have to hire a food technologist to prepare their menus! To prove their point, they presented a menu from one of the local restaurants as it currently was, and another of the same menu but listing all of the chemicals in each entrée. They did our homework for us! The most notable entrée was their turkey salad sandwich. It had *11 typewritten lines* listing the chemicals that were in it! In a simple turkey salad sandwich!

Unfortunately, the members of both houses caved in under the pressure from our prestigious opponents, and the bill did not pass. Nonetheless, we did make our point. And I believe that someday, a similar bill will pass in every state.

Some Chemicals in our foods:

Sprouting inhibitors
It used to be that whenever you bought potatoes, you could tell the approximate age of the spuds by the size and extent of the growth of the eyes. However, some years ago it became apparent that some potatoes never sprouted from their "eyes." Some investigation into this phenomenon brought out the fact that many growers, probably due to demand from distributors, now treat the potatoes with a growth-inhibiting chemical. This may be done after harvest, *or before.*

When I first learned of this, the chemical was called "Sprout Nip" and it works like this: Sometime before harvest, when the potato foliage is still green, the farmer sprays the field with the chemical. The foliage accepts the chemical and actually takes it into the plant itself and then down *into* the tubers. In essence, what this means is that when you eat the potato you are eating the chemical as part of the potato. Apparently the chemical is not in itself seriously toxic, but as we mentioned above, we may not be dealing with "short term" effects. Rather, we might need to consider "long term effects" or even possibly the interaction of this chemical with another of the 4,999 chemicals in our food supply.

In addition to "Sprout Nip", some of the other products used are "Royal MH-30; Royal MH-30 Xtra; "Sprout Stop"; Sprout Stop 80 WS. Aside from the fancy names used for the benefit of the farmers, Maleic hydrazide and chlorpropham (CIPC) are the compounds most commonly used as sprout inhibitors in these products. 11 These chemicals are also used to prevent volunteer growth the following season of the potatoes that have been left in the field, very possibly contaminating the soil and ground water.

Systemic insecticides and fungicides

Another source of chemicals in our food first came to my attention when I was reading a farm journal some years ago. There was an advertisement that caught my eye. The headline read "One Bite and the Insect Dies." Reading further I learned about the introduction and use of systemic insecticides. This type of insecticide is either applied to the foliage or directed toward the roots. The insecticide is absorbed into the plant and travels with the plant sap to all parts of the plant. The insects that feed on the plant take in this chemical and simply die.12

Could this possibly have an effect on us?

The manufacturers claim the following: "The benefits of using systemic insecticides plants include:

(1) plants are continuously protected throughout most of the growing season without the need for repeat applications

(2) these insecticides are not susceptible to ultraviolet light degradation or "wash off" during watering,

(3) there is less unsightly residue on foliage or flowers, and

(4) harmful effects to workers and customers are minimal.

Once again, I find this disconcerting because they are in essence admitting that there *are* some harmful effects on workers and consumers. 13 Other problems stated are that these chemicals may more than likely enter the ground water, and that continued use will eventually result in resistant genotypes. 14 In other words, they will encourage the reproduction of insects that are resistant to insecticides. Some examples of these systemic products are as follows: aba-mectin (Avid), pyriproxyfen (Distance), chlorfenapyr (Pylon), spinosad (Conserve), and acephate (Orthene).

I might mention that systemic chemicals are also being used to control plant viruses. 15 The immediate harm is probably the least of our worries; what frightens me is the potential for long-term toxicity and the potential for interaction with other chemicals in our diets. And as mentioned above, even if the target plant is a shrub or tree, or flowers, my fear would center on the contamination of the ground water. By the very admission of its producers most of these products are extremely toxic to all animals. 16,17

I'm sure that you are getting the point, and rather than to belabor that point, suffice it to say that many of our foods are laden with chemicals. It is argued that they are necessary in order to supply our population with safe and attractive food. But how far should the producers go with these chemicals? Should you the consumer know something about it so you can make your own choices? I say yes!

However, there is one choice in my mind that is unacceptable, and that is to throw up your hands and say, "I give up, there's nothing safe left to eat!" There is plenty to choose from. Furthermore, it is important to demand quality foods and to back that up by purchasing them, which will encourage the producers toward more organic, natural foods. And, do you know what? It's working! Look around – we are seeing more and more "natural foods" on the market than ever before.

REFERENCES FOOD ADDITIVES

1. http://vm.cfsan.fda.gov/~dms/eafus.html
2. http://www.access.gpo.gov/nara/cfr/waisidx_01/21cfrv3_01.html
3. http://frwebgate1.access.gpo.gov/cgi-bin/waisgate.cgi?WAIS docID=77599624838+4+0+0&WAISaction=retrieve
4. http://frwebgate2.access.gpo.gov/cgi-bin/waisgate.cgi?WAIS docID=778131249060+2+0+0&WAISaction=retrieve
5. http://frwebgate4.access.gpo.gov/cgi-bin/waisgate.cgi?WAIS docID=75892623794+9+0+0&WAISaction=retrieve
6. http://www.cspinet.org/reports/chemcuisine.htm
7. http://vm.cfsan.fda.gov/~dms/opa-cg8.html
8. http://www.foodriskclearinghouse.umd.edu/food_and_color_additives.cfm#toppage
9. http://frwebgate1.access.gpo.gov/cgi-bin/waisgate.cgi?WAIS docID=75767514336+5+0+0&WAISaction=retrieve
10. http://www.extension.umn.edu/distribution/nutrition/DJ0974.html
11. http://www.mainepotatopestguide.com/potatosproutinhibitors.asp
12. http://www.mobot.org/gardeninghelp/hortline/messages/3145.shtml
13. http://www.ag.uiuc.edu/cespubs/hyg/html/200220e.html
14. http://www.ag.uiuc.edu/cespubs/hyg/html/200220e.html
15. http://potatovariety.oregonstate.edu/Systemics.htm
16. http://www.colostate.edu/Depts/IPM/ento/j521fd.html
17. http://www.colostate.edu/Depts/IPM/ento/j511e.html

6.

MENTAL AND EMOTIONAL ILLNESS

Abstract

For many years it was thought that mental illness was a manifestation of the mind related to previous experiences, incorrect thinking and various emotional traumata.

Although there is something to be said about those concepts, it is now becoming more and more apparent that many neurosis and psychoses are the result of imbalanced brain chemistry. Indeed, the brain must have very specific chemical balances in order to function properly. Sometimes these imbalances are the result of genetics and perhaps even congenital problems. But lately we are beginning to recognize that the chemistry of the brain is affected by the chemistry we put into our bodies in the form of nutrition. In this chapter we discuss many of these nutritional aspects and how we can prevent them.

When someone contracts measles, it is expressed outwardly on the skin as tiny red bumps called macules. A case of mumps is expressed by a swelling of the parotid glands of the neck. Multiple sclerosis is expressed by muscle weakness, loss of balance, and speech and visual disturbances.

Even minor sub-acute nutritional deficiency diseases are expressed outwardly in some manner. A deficiency of vitamin A will cause keratosis pilaris, a roughness of the skin, and a thickening of the sclera of the eyes. The point is that with each disease, there is an outward expression. So it is also with chemical and nutritional deficiencies of the brain. But the outward expression will not be something that can be seen, but rather will be expressed as psychological and emotional problems.

The brain chemistry must remain within certain parameters in order to function normally. If these brain chemicals are deficient, or not properly balanced, the outward expression will be the neuroses and psychoses that we recognize as mental and emotional illness. Although for many years the common approach to correcting mental and emotional illness has been various types of psychotherapy, it is becoming increasingly more obvious that these disorders are indeed problems involving biochemical imbalances in the brain.

In psychiatry, pharmaceutical drugs are used to relax a patient, reduce depression, and in general, to alter behavior. However, except for certain genetic disorders, it is becoming ever more obvious that mental and emotional illness can be treated or even prevented with proper nutrition.

In other words, nutritional deficiencies lead to chemical imbalances that in turn lead to altered function, and eventually, aberrant behavior. Chemical imbalances of the brain can be caused by several factors:

Hypoglycemia (low blood sugar)
Toxemia from insufficient vitamin B
Hypoxia (the lack of sufficient oxygen)
Imbalances or deficiencies of neurotransmitters such as serotonin and acetylcholine.

So, let's go through each, one by one to explore these concepts.

1. **Hypoglycemia,** or low blood sugar, is a condition that has stirred considerable controversy in the past several decades. Some physicians even fail to acknowledge its existence. A number of books and studies however have proven to the satisfaction of many that it is a condition that must be considered. 1, 2

First, all carbohydrates that we eat, whether starches or sugars, enter our circulating blood as the simple sugar "glucose." This is the principal food energy source for our bodies. It circulates in our blood as glucose. Bear in mind that glucose is also the brain's main source of energy.

As with other factors in the body, there is a range of normalcy and health for all body chemicals. In the circulating blood, the normal range for glucose is between 80 and 120 mg % (mg per 100 liters of blood). After a typical meal it is not uncommon for the blood sugar to rise even as high as 200 mg %. But if the blood sugar remains above 140 mg for any great period of time, then high blood sugar or hyperglycemia, commonly called diabetes, is present.

It works like this: after a meal high in carbohydrates, the blood sugar rises. When it reaches a certain point, a trigger mechanism (probably within the brain) causes the release of insulin. It is the job of insulin to take excess sugar out of the blood and to cause it to be stored in body tissues, such as the liver and muscles, thus bringing the blood sugar back into the normal range. I should mention here that from the experience with many cases I have found that a normal person can create hypoglycemia problems by submitting this "trigger mechanism" to frequent stimulation, i.e., by eating excessive amounts of sugar or caffeine. When this occurs it seems to sensitize this trigger. Thus, the more the trigger gets sensitized, the greater the release of insulin, and the lower the hypoglycemia goes. The problem of hypoglycemia arises because of one major factor. The human body was never meant to handle the effects of large amounts of sugar (or caffeine, but that's another discussion!).

The response to a deluge of sugar is an overreaction by the body, which causes the dumping of a huge amount of insulin, far and above what is needed to bring the blood sugar to its normal range. The result of the excess insulin is to cause the blood sugar to drop way below normal, bringing the body into a state of "hypoglycemia" or low blood sugar. In other words eating large amounts of sugar can cause low blood sugar 3

As mentioned above, the brain is very sensitive to chemical imbalances, including a drop of glucose (blood sugar) it's main source of energy.. A low level of glucose is essentially incompatible with normal brain function, and a number of symptoms can occur. Various texts list the following symptoms associated with low blood sugar: 3, 4

HUNGER	ARGUEMENTIVENESS
WEAKNESS	CRYING SPELLS
FATIGUE	CONFUSION
ANXIETY	TREMULOUSNESS
NERVOUSNESS	INCOORDINATION FOR FINE MOVEMENTS
IRRITABILITY	INABILITY TO CONCENTRATE
ANGER	HEADACHE
DEPRESSION	SUICIDE

From actual clinical experience of hundreds of cases, I can honestly say that no two cases are alike. Different people have different reactions to differing extents.

When testing for hypoglycemia, a single blood test is almost totally worthless. It is normally given in the morning, on an empty stomach, If the results indicate exceptionally high glucose levels, it is rather certain that there is a presence of diabetes to some degree. But one fasting sample will not point out what kind of reaction a person might have after the intake of a large amount of sugar. The typical glucose tolerance test to determine diabetes should be continued for at least three hours, but preferably for six hours. 5

To get a proper diagnosis for hypoglycemia, the test should be a 6-hour glucose tolerance test given as follows: 6 The patient fasts overnight. At the lab in the morning, a blood sample is taken before anything is eaten. The patient is then given a large glass of sugar water to drink. Thereafter, a blood sample is taken every 1/2 hour.

Examples of several 6 hour glucose tolerance tests :

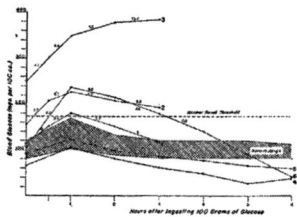

1. A mild case of diabetes.
2. Moderately severe diabetes
3. Extremely severe diabetes
4. Manifest hyperinsulinism. (This patient has severe hypoglycemia)
5. Moderate hypoglycemia
6. Unusual hypoglycemia that would not show up in a 3 hour test.

No two graphs I have ever seen have been the same. To be very frank, some people have very little reaction from the consumption of sugar at all. It is a very individual thing. Early in my career, while I was still in professional school, I worked as a dormitory supervisor at The Youth House for Boys, a facility for the temporary detention of juvenile delinquents in New York City. During that time, I had contact with many hundreds of boys of varying ages. Each week, the facility had visiting hours where families were allowed to see the children and to bring them "goodies." It soon became vividly apparent that after the parents left, the boys would, as the expression goes, be "bouncing off the walls!" At that time, I began studying and accumulating research relating to this aberrant behavior. The result was my first published study entitled, "The Nutritive Factors in Delinquency." 7 This study outlined the reactions in children caused by low blood sugar, cerebral hypoxia and cerebral toxemia.

To explain briefly, a high intake of sugar (in some people) causes a resultant hypoglycemia. The drop in blood sugar starves the brain cells of sufficient glucose to function normally. At the same time, in order for the cells to change the sugar into energy, they need the B vitamins as co-enzymes (organic catalysts). If that same individual is deficient in these vitamins, there will be an accumulation of intermediary carbohydrate breakdown products in the brain, principally pyruvic acid. Hence, in a B vitamin deficiency, pyruvic acid accumulates in the brain, which in itself is toxic to brain cells. The presence of pyruvic acid also reduces the "oxygen saturation potential" of the brain tissues, causing a reduced oxygen condition called hypoxia. This results in a triple condition of hypoglycemia, toxemia and hypoxia of the brain cells. Of these three conditions, I'm not sure which has the greater effect on the emotional problems, or indeed if they must all be present to cause the aberrant behavior.

At one time in my practice, I worked with a psychologist friend who monitored his wife during an entire 6-hour glucose tolerance test. When comparing his notes of her reactions and my charted graph of her hypoglycemia, we discovered that the greatest emotional expressions were not so much when the hypoglycemia was in its lowest stages, but more so as the glucose levels were dropping!

Throughout the years of my practice I have had the opportunity to work with hundreds of hypoglycemic patients, and have found that this condition can indeed cause many problems if unchecked and misunderstood. From the symptoms mentioned above, to kicking and thrashing in bed at night, to personality changes, many reactions are classic.

Let's look at just a few scenarios:

Auto accidents – You will note from highway statistics that more accidents on highways and freeways occur during the drive home in the evening. This has been commonly attributed to the fatigue at the end of the workday. But I maintain that hypoglycemia is also greatly involved. For example, most people lunch around noon, and then around mid-afternoon they take a coffee break. (Let's talk about coffee later.) This may be accompanied by a donut or other "goodie" and perhaps sugar in the coffee. This combination causes a temporary rise in the blood sugar, with the resultant severe drop 1/2 - 1 hour later – right during the drive home. What were some of the symptoms listed above? *"Depression, irritability, anxiety, incoordination for fine movements..."* Put those together in a situation of highway traffic, add some male machismo and the results can be tragic.

Divorce – I guess it would be bad enough if one member of the relationship suffered from *depression, irritability, nervousness and anger*, but if both people contribute these difficult symptoms, I can imagine some very volatile arguments that could very well contribute to eventual divorce.

Juvenile delinquency – According to published findings by physician Joseph Wilder, MD, of New York, a child in a state of hypoglycemia, " ... may be neurotic, psychopathic, or have criminal tendencies, and may be subject to anxiety, running away tendencies, aggressiveness, a blind urge to activity and destructiveness with impairment of moral sensibilities like shame." 8 Dr. Wilder's observations were tested in Argentina by researchers N. Rojas and A.F. Sanchi. They actually tested the blood sugar levels of apprehended delinquents and of 129 delinquents examined, 48 cases showed blood sugar levels less than 75 mg %. In 64 cases the blood sugar was between 75 and 90 mg %. One individual tested as low as 38 mg %. In only 13 cases was the blood sugar within the normal range. 9

In the early 1980s Alexander Schauss went on to further examine the effects of sugar on juvenile delinquents. In his published findings he reported that a multitude of double blind, crossover studies were done throughout the U.S. in detention units involving more than 10,000 juveniles. It was found that the incidence of antisocial behavior was reduced consistently between 36% and 59% when sugar was omitted from their diets. 10

I'm sure that with a little imagination you can understand other idiosyncratic behaviors and scenarios in yourself and others relating to hypoglycemia. But before we leave the subject I must bring to your attention the effects of coffee on this condition. Caffeine in itself has a remarkable effect on the human system. Specifically, caffeine causes a release of stored glycogen (sugar) from the liver. However, the result is not always casual or subtle. 11 The caffeine from one cup of coffee is said to be 80 – 135 mg. 12 This could release the approximate amount of sugar as would be found in one to two candy bars. If you happen to be "hooked" on cola drinks, the prognosis is not much better. Many cola drinks can deliver as much as 40 – 71 mg. of caffeine from one 12-ounce can. 13 That's the reason why a cup of coffee or cola drinks gives you a "lift." But, this is not a healthy way to give yourself a boost of energy. If you yield to the common notion that a candy bar or a cup of coffee is the solution as you run short of energy during the day, the eventual results could be disastrous. Each time you succumb to a sugary, caffeine laden snack, you further sensitize the insulin release trigger, thereby causing increasingly greater amounts of insulin to be secreted, which in turn can cause the hypoglycemic events to become more profound with ever greater symptoms. I challenge you to begin to notice in yourself and others around you the escalating need to use coffee throughout the day.

2. Toxemia from Insufficient vitamin B
As mentioned above, the glucose in our blood is used as the prime energy source for all of our tissues. But the glucose has

to be changed into energy within each cell. This occurs as the result of a series of reactions that take place with the glucose. In biochemistry, this is called the "citric acid cycle" during which the glucose is changed into different chemicals. Some of the most important stages it goes through are as follows:

GLUCOSE → PYRUVIC ACID → ACETYL PHOSPHATE → – ACETIC ACID = *ENERGY* + WATER + CARBON DIOXIDE 14

It seems simple enough to make the assumption that the chemical reaction just happens. But the important thing in chemistry is that these reactions need catalysts in order to proceed from one stage to the next. In organic chemistry, these catalysts are called enzymes and co-enzymes. *The co-enzymes needed in this energy release from glucose are the B vitamins.* It is interesting to note also that the symptoms given for a B vitamin deficiency are the same as those for hypoglycemia, i.e., depression, irritability, anxiety, uncertainty of memory, etc. 15 If these vitamins are not available at the specific time, the reaction may be interrupted at an intermediate stage thus allowing pyruvic acid, the apparent worst culprit, to accumulate within the tissue spaces, acting as a toxin to the cells. Within the muscles the effect is not as great as it is in the brain where it can cause great distress. 16 It should also be noted that a high carbohydrate diet in itself increases the need for the B vitamins. 17, 18

If sugar and carbohydrates can be implicated in this problem, then refined carbohydrates can be said to greatly exaggerate it. The reason for this is that in the refining of almost all of the common carbohydrate foods, most of the inherent B vitamins are removed.

For example, when wheat is refined into white flour, the bran and germ, the main sources of the B vitamins, are removed. When brown rice is polished to make white rice, the polishings,

which are the main source of the B vitamins, are removed.
When sugar cane is refined to make white sugar, the B vitamin-
rich molasses is removed. In other words, B vitamins, which are
necessary to release energy from the basic carbohydrates, are
naturally present in these foods until we intentionally refine
them away.

3. Hypoxia (insufficient oxygen)

The accumulation of the toxic intermediary products of
carbohydrate metabolism within the brain results in decreased
oxygen saturation. In other words, the oxygen is unable to achieve
the proper concentration within the tissues. Nathan Masor,
M.D., described the consequences as follows: "The arterial
blood saturation of oxygen to the brain should be well over 90
percent for proper psychic functioning. In terms of percentage,
a reduction to 85 percent saturation decreases the ability for
fine concentration and reduces muscular coordination. Further
reduction to 74 percent leads to faulty judgement and emotional
lability. Still further reduction leads to progressive depression
of the central nervous system." 19

4. Imbalances and deficiencies of neurotransmitters such serotonin, acetylcholine and other nutritional factors.

It seems that we are in the early stages of our understanding
of the nutritional needs for proper psychic functioning as
combined with the influence of individual genetics. For example
it is apparent from Roger Williams' work with biochemical
individuality that genetics counts a great deal when we realize
that nutrients are absorbed differently even in brothers and
sisters within the same family. 15 Why this is so is not fully
understood. My feeling is that, as we understand the nutrients
needed for proper brain and psychic functioning and can
recognize the outward signs of malfunction, we might really
be dealing with simply a nutritional deficiency, or perhaps an
inability for that person to absorb those vital nutrients. 20

Amino acid deficiencies

Except for the skeletal system, almost all of the other tissues of our bodies are protein, and the building blocks of proteins are the amino acids. Of the several hundred amino acids found in nature, about 40 – 50 are found in human blood. Eight of those are considered in human nutrition as "essential" because although the human body is able to change or combine parts of amino acids with other amino acids to fill all jobs within the body, it cannot build any of those eight! They must be taken in specifically from the diet. What's more, some studies suggest that those eight essential amino acids must be on hand at the same time in order to synthesize all of the other needs. 25 This means that they must be taken at the same meal!

Several specific amino acids however seem to be needed for very specific jobs within the brain. In a published paper that I wrote several years ago, I mentioned specific amino acids that are implicated in psychiatric behaviors. 26

Tryptophan, tyrosine & phenylalanine are several amino acids directly involved as precursors of important "neurotransmitters" within the nervous system. The most important of these neurotransmitters is called serotonin. Although tryptophan is probably the chief amino acid in creating serotonin, both tyrosine and phenylalanine are also involved. Neurotransmitters are responsible for transmitting impulses across nerve junctions, without which the nerve system would cease to function.

Tryptophan, tyrosine and phenylalanine are vital in human nutrition. Because of their importance as neurotransmitters, several conditions have been connected with their deficiency. The most important of these are "acute manic conditions" and depression. In many double blind studies, these nutrients have proven invaluable in treating those conditions. 27, 28, 29, 30

Although studies have thusfar indicated that these three amino acids are extremely important with regard to emotional health, in the future others may be found equally important. Moreover, as with the B complex vitamins, which work synergistically together, it is my contention that the amino acids may also function in a similar way. Hence taking singular synthetic amino acids may not function as well as consuming a food that contains all of the important amino acids naturally.

Of the three amino acids mentioned above, tryptophan and phenylalanine are considered "essential" amino acids. Foods that contain all eight of the essential amino acids are called complete proteins. In general, animal protein such as meat, fish, dairy products and eggs are complete while vegetable protein is typically incomplete. This is not to say that one vegetable containing several of these amino acids cannot be complemented by another containing the rest. Bear in mind however, as mentioned above, in order to complement each other as such, they must be consumed at the same meal. One specific book deals with this subject completely. Diet for a Small Planet, by Frances Moore Lappe, offers multiple suggestions for combining vegetable proteins.

We have much to learn about the functioning of the human brain, however, and it is my contention that diet will hold the key to many of our mental and emotional problems.

Once again my recommendation is to aim for complete and balanced nutrition from natural sources.

In addition to understanding the concepts listed above, we are finding that other nutritional factors are equally as important.

Minerals
Several minerals have been recognized as important to mental health.

Chromium is significant because it is involved as a part of what is called the glucose tolerance factor, which is an organic complex of chromium with dinicotino-glutathione. Whether we are dealing with hyperglycemia (diabetes) or hypoglycemia (low blood sugar), the glucose tolerance factor is instrumental in normalizing the blood sugar. Hence chromium would be important in both syndromes. 21, 22

The glucose tolerance factor can be purchased as such, or it can be assembled within the body if the three important nutrients chromium, nicotinic acid, and glutathione are available.

Zinc appears to have a profound effect on brain development, function, and behavior. During pre- and postnatal development of the brain, even moderate deficiencies of zinc appear to be vitally significant. Zinc deficiency in animal studies has been associated with abnormal EEG activity, irritability, mood changes, abnormal visual behavior, impaired problem solving, long-term memory loss, and increased risk for Alzheimer's disease, schizophrenia and epilepsy. 23

Magnesium was mentioned in a report from the Bio-behavioral Psychiatry Institute in Great Neck, New York, which acknowledged that there are nutritional components in the biological aspect of aberrant behavior as seen in both animal and human studies. The researchers found that the mineral magnesium is a vital component in preventing aggressiveness. 24

REFERENCES – MENTAL AND EMOTIONAL ILLNESS

1. Body Mind and Sugar. E.M. Abrahamson and A.W. Pizet; Henry Holt and Company. N.Y. 1959.
2. Low Blood Sugar and You. Carlton Fredericks and Herman goodman. Constellation International N.Y. 1969.

3. Body Mind and Sugar ; p. 62, 63

4. Low Blood Sugar and You; pp. 32,33

5. MEDLINEplus Medical Encyclopedia: Glucose tolerance test.

6. Body Mind and Sugar; p. 55.

7. Trapani F J, The Nutritive Factors in Delinquency; National Chiropratic Association Journal. March 1961.

8. Joseph Wilder M.D., N.Y. The Nervous Child. April 1943,44.

9. N. Rojas; A.F. Sanchi; Archives of Legal Medicine. Vol. 11, 1941. 29.

10. Alexander Schauss; Nutrition and Social Behavior. Yearbook of Nutritional Medicine. 1984-85.

11. Body Mind and Sugar; pp. 65,66.

12. Bunker and McWilliams in J. Am. Diet. 74:28-32, 1979:

13 National Soft Drink Association; Courtesy of the Seven-Up Company

14 Kleiner and Orten, Human Biochemistry; C.V. MosbyCo.., St. Louis. 1958 320.

15 Roger J. Williams. Biochemical Individuality, John Wiley and Sons, Inc. N.Y.1956 203, 204.

16 Best and Taylor. Physiological Basis of Medical Practice. Third Edition. 1943. 1078.

17 Kleiner and Orten; op cit.No.3, 313. 318.

18 Best and Taylor; op.cit.No.2.1078, 1079.

19 Nathan Masor, M.D. The New Psychiatry. Philosophical Press, N.Y. p 20.

20 Blom W. van den Berg G, Huijmans J: Successful Nicotinamide treatment in an autosomal dominant behavioral and psychiatric disorder.J Inh Met D 1985: 8: 107,108

21 Richard A. Anderson. PhD; The Role of Chromium in the Control of High and Low Blood Sugar. The Nutrition Report, Health Media of America Vol. 6 No. 6.June 1988.

22 Anderson R, Polansky M, Bryden N, et al: Effects of supplemental chromium on patients with symptoms of reactive hypoglycemia. Metabolism 1987; 36: 351-355.

23 J.C. Wallwork. Prog Food Nutr Sci. 1987; 11:203-247.

24 Yaryura-Tobias J; Biological aspects of aggressive behavior. Int. J. Neurs 1987;32:890.

25 Applied Trophology. Standard Process Laboratories, Vol. 8 No. 11 Nov.1964.

26 Trapani, F J. Singular Effects of the Amino Acids.,WCA Journal Jan. 1983.

27 Russ M, Ackerman S, Banay-SchwartzM, et al: Plasma Tryptophan to large neutral amino acid ratios in depressed and normal subjects. J Affect D 1990;19:9-14.

28 Chouinard G,Young S,Annable L,:A controlled clinical trialof L-tryptophan in acute mania. Biol.Psychi 1985;20:546-557.

29 Moller S: Tryptophan and tyrosine ratios to neutral amino acids in relation to therapeutic response in depressed patients. Int J Neurs 1987:32:570-571.

30 Sabelli H, Fawcell J, Gusofsky F, et al: Clinical studies on the phenylethylamine hypothesis of affective disorder: Urine and blood phenylacetic acid and phenylalanine dietary supplements. J Clin Psy 1986;47:66-70.

7.

CARDIOVASCULAR DISEASE

Abstract

*B*y far, the leading cause of death among the industrialized nations is cardiovascular disease. However, I feel that the death rate from this disease can be reduced by 80% with just a few changes to our diets. We have at our disposal certain food supplements that have a profound effect on prevention of this disease.

In this chapter you will begin to understand the meaning of such words as "plaque", "atherosclerosis" "platelet aggregation" "angina pectoris" and much more. You will find out why the Greenland Eskimo who have the highest intake of fat in their diet have the lowest coronary disease rate in the world.

In terms of meaningful advice, this might be the most important chapter for saving your life, or the lives of your loved ones.

To begin with, you should have some knowledge about just what the cardiovascular system is so let's start there. Each of us is composed of about three trillion cells, each of which requires maintenance. Each cell needs food and oxygen, and each cell needs to get rid of waste products like carbon dioxide and the byproducts of metabolism. The cells themselves cannot move, so it is the job of the circulatory system to facilitate the jobs of nourishment and cleansing.

The hemoglobin in the red blood cells picks up oxygen as it travels through the lungs and brings it to each cell. The hemoglobin also picks up the carbon dioxide from the cells and brings it back to the lungs where it is exhaled. In similar manner. The liquid of the blood, called plasma, carries nutrients to each cell, and carries the wastes away to the kidneys to be processed for excretion. For all this to happen, the blood must be in constant motion. The heart is the pump that maintains continuous circulation of the blood.

The heart itself is comprised of four chambers that direct the blood through the arteries to the cells of the body and to the lungs. The heart is a muscle, but unlike other muscles, it begins working before birth and does not stop until death. Also unlike other muscles, the only rest it gets is between beats. But just like other muscles of the body, it must have oxygen and nutrients. These it receives via the coronary arteries that bring the blood with its essential nutrients and oxygen back to the heart muscle itself.

The term "cardiovascular" is a compound word that refers to two systems, the heart (cardio) and the blood vessels (vascular) systems. Because cardiovascular disease (CVD) is commonly thought of as a condition involving only the heart, it is important that we include here a discussion of "stroke" since it also involves pathology of the vascular system, but within the brain.

CVD is the nation's leading killer for both men and women and among all racial and ethnic groups. Nearly one million Americans die of CVD each year, which adds up to about 42 percent of all deaths in the United States. 1 Statistically it costs our nation around $300 billion dollars each year in health expenditures and lost productivity. It is our nation's leading health problem!

Let's establish a glossary of words pertaining to this subject:

CAD – Coronary Artery Disease – when the coronary arteries become clogged with plaque

Plaque – an accumulation of cholesterol and other materials on the inner lining of blood vessels, which make the lumen or opening narrower.

Atherosclerosis – the condition wherein an artery or arteriole becomes clogged with plaque, lessening and slowing the flow of blood within it

Platelets – those tiny bodies within circulating blood that contain blood clotting chemicals

Platelet aggregation – the clumping together of platelets to form a clot

Plaque fragmentation (thromboembolus) – a piece of plaque breaking loose into the general blood circulation

Embolus – anything circulating in the blood that doesn't belong there

Infarct – when a clot or fragment of plaque clogs an artery or arteriole blocking blood flow to the tissues beyond

Myocardial infarction – when the infarct is in the heart muscle itself

Angina pectoris – when plaque develops within the coronary vessels preventing them from carrying sufficient blood to the heart muscle itself causing reflexive pain to the pectoralis muscle on the left side

Vasospasm – spasm of the muscular walls of the artery itself, reducing or stopping the flow of blood within

Variant angina – a condition involving vasospasm of the coronary arteries

Stroke – general term for three separate events involving blood circulation to and within the brain (described below)

Arteriosclerosis – a hardening of the muscular walls of an artery with the deposition of calcium therein

Thrombogenesis – the genesis or development of any type of clot in the circulating blood

Thromboxane – a chemical found within the platelets that causes platelet clumping and also constricts the diameter of a blood vessel

Prostacyclin – a chemical secreted from the blood vessel walls that dissolves clots and causes enlargement of the vessel diameter

Now, let's begin with a discussion of the most significant types of cardiovascular disease and stroke:

First is atherosclerosis, a condition where there is an accumulation of plaque within the blood vessels.

Second is the formation of blood clots within the circulating blood.

Third is a condition called "variant angina."

When dealing with stroke, there are similar problems:

First, there is the possibility of a blood vessel actually bursting – this causes bleeding into the tissue spaces and a pooling of the blood within the brain.

Second, as with the heart, there can be blockage of an artery by a clot.

Third, there can be a similar condition as mentioned above in variant angina where an artery goes into spasm not allowing blood to pass through.

The important thing in attempting to understand atherosclerosis is to determine just what causes the accumulation of plaque. This condition does not happen overnight, but takes years to develop. In fact, during autopsies performed on young soldiers during the Korean and Vietnam wars, these men were shown to have well developed atherosclerotic lesions within their arteries, indicating that the problem of plaque accumulation, at least in Americans, begins early in life. 2, 3

The cause of the development of atherosclerosis is now becoming very clear. But the mechanism of its occurrence and the cause of its occurrence are both important. In other words, how it happens and why it happens are two different things. The mechanism of atherosclerosis starts with inflammation or an injury on the inner arterial wall. The actual cause of this situation is not clearly understood: some think that the main problem is inflammation caused by a chemical called "homocysteine" and other researchers think that it is a problem called "monoclonal proliferation" which is caused by "free radicals." Homocysteine is actually an amino acid produced from the metabolism of the amino acid called methionine. If methionine is metabolized in the absence of vitamin B6 and folic acid, it forms the chemical homocysteine, which has been found in high concentrations in people with atherosclerosis. Methionine happens to be present in high concentrations in meat, and hence meat eaters require more vitamin B than non-meat eaters. Circulating blood products, including platelets and fibrin, deposit on the injury or inflammation. Over time, there is an accumulation of fatty molecules, particularly cholesterol, over the injured site. This process produces organized scarred lesions or plaques. These plaques can enlarge into the lumen (tubular cavity) and partially obstruct the vessel, thus diminishing blood supply to the tissues that it feeds. 4

When the coronary vessels that feed the heart have accumulations of plaque, the flow of oxygen and nutrients to the heart muscle itself is restricted, resulting in coronary heart disease. As part of the symptoms, the pectoral muscle (the chest muscle) on the left side expresses pain. That is why the condition is called angina (meaning a spasmodic attack of pain) pectoris (in the pectoral muscle). (In early stages, the pain may be very mild.)

Let's create a scenario: a man in whom plaque has been slowly accumulating over the years is taking a walk. He comes to a wide street and decides to cross. As he begins crossing he spots a truck bearing down on him and is forced to run the rest of the way to the other side. The muscles in his legs require extra blood and his lungs demand more air, causing the heart to beat faster to supply these needs. Even though the heart beats faster, the blockage caused by the plaque does not allow the blood going through the coronary arteries to get into the heart muscle fast enough. Without sufficient oxygen the heart expresses pain in the chest muscles. The man grabs his chest and when he gets to the other side, he sits down on the curb. The heart eventually slows down, demanding less oxygen. The insufficient blood supply is then enough to satisfy its resting pulse and pain ceases. If the man had been seeing a doctor for his condition, he might have had some nitroglycerin pills in his pocket which could have given him immediate relief since they have a specific action to dilate or open the coronary arteries temporarily.

Although technically atherosclerosis is correctly listed as a CVD statistic, the truth of the matter is that only about 15,000 people in the United States (less than 1percent of all deaths, 1999 statistics) actually die from atherosclerosis annually. This is not the big killer! When we discuss the effects of clots below, you will see that plaque can cause the formation of blood clots, which is the more dangerous part of the story.

Bear in mind that I'm not stating that plaque is not a problem; it is – hence the development of medical procedures such as balloon angioplasty and rotoablation. The most recent and apparently the most successful procedure is bypass surgery, where the blocked arteries are removed and other vessels are spliced into their place.

My feeling has always been to ask the question, "Why"? Why does this plaque develop? What causes it to develop? Let's try to answer those questions now.

Unfortunately, one substance has been incorrectly isolated as the root cause of all of our heart problems, and hence, "cholesterol" has become a buzzword of fear. Even though cholesterol is a major part of the substance of plaque itself, it is inaccurate to identify it as the cause of cardiovascular disease.

So, let's talk about this substance called cholesterol, which is a vital ingredient of our chemical makeup.

It is needed for hormone production.

It is essential for brain and nerve development.

It is the starting material from which the liver produces bile acids.

It is a key substance in the walls of every cell in our body.

In the skin, it changes to vitamin D with the radiation of sunshine.

In fact, the liver produces cholesterol for all of these functions. You've heard that we should restrict or limit intake of foods that contain cholesterol, but in all except a few individuals who have a genetic defect, the body will control the amount of cholesterol produced. The more cholesterol consumed through diet, the less the liver produces, and vice versa.

Cholesterol is a multifaceted substance comprised of several factors: high-density lipoprotein (HDL), intermediate density lipoprotein (IDL), low-density lipoprotein (LDL) and very low-density lipoprotein (VLDL). Of these four, only HDL and LDL are of prime importance to our discussion.

The LDL molecule is responsible for transporting organic compounds called lipids from the liver to the body. The HDL molecule is responsible for transporting these lipids from the cells of the body back to the liver for destruction in order to maintain a balance within the tissues.

We can say therefore that the HDL is a good factor because it diminishes the amount of total accumulated cholesterol by eliminating it where it is not needed, even from within the arteries themselves. And the LDL is the bad factor because it has the ability of depositing cholesterol in various parts of the body. This is the "stuff" that becomes part of the offending plaque that is deposited, occluding the arteries. Yet, that is not the final word. Now we must learn what increases and decreases the good and the bad factors in cholesterol.

One way LDL is increased in the body is through a high fat diet. Fat can be in a solid or liquid form (oil). Eating lots of fat is not a good idea, especially solid fats, which tend to increase the LDL levels. But worse yet is eating processed oils that have been hydrogenated. These oils are processed by saturating the molecules with hydrogen to make them more solid and to increase their "shelf life," but during the hydrogenation process, "trans" fats are created that tend not only increase the LDL, but to decrease the HDL. This is the process by which margarine and most peanut butters are produced.

These harmful "trans" fats are found in products like margarine, shortening, commercially baked foods, the commercial oils used to make French fries and other fast foods, and in certain "hydrogenated" peanut butter. These are major culprits. One problem with trans fat is that food companies are not required to list it on nutrition labels so consumers have no way of knowing how much trans fat is in the food they are eating. Further, there is no safety limit recommended for the daily intake of trans fat. The Food and Drug Administration (FDA) has only said "intake of trans fats should be as low as possible." 5, 6, 7

Even though the LDL is a contributing factor in heart disease, it must first undergo peroxidation before it contributes to plaque. In chemical terms, peroxidation is the loss of electrons. In common terms, peroxidation would be akin to the fat becoming rancid within our bodies. In order to prevent this, a constant supply of "antioxidants" should always be present. In 1993 U.S. News and World Report carried a story citing a study reported in the New England Journal of Medicine. The study involved 87,245 nurses and 39,910 doctors who took a daily dose

100 I.U. of vitamin E (a powerful antioxidant). The findings indicated that those who took the vitamin E "had significantly fewer heart attacks and arterial problems than those who didn't take the supplements. In fact, the statistics indicate 42 percent fewer heart attacks! The theory is that vitamin E inhibits the ability of LDL, the so-called bad cholesterol, to become plaque and to clog arteries." 9

The above study followed many other related studies that suggested the importance of preventing the peroxidation of the LDL cholesterol with vitamin E and also the mineral selenium. 10,11,12

Vitamin E is so important in preventing heart disease that the World Health Organization sponsored a study to investigate this concept. The results were so profound that the conclusions in the study state that a low level of vitamin E is the key risk factor in death from coronary artery disease ‾ more significant than high cholesterol, elevated blood pressure, or smoking. In fact, low levels of vitamin E can be used as a predictor of heart disease, since a finding of low vitamin E predicted ischemic heart disease mortality in 62 percent of the cases. 13 This comprehensive study involved subjects from 10 countries.

It seems quite clear that LDL will not harm you if you take sufficient antioxidants such as vitamin E and selenium. With this array of knowledgeable and authentic studies, why do we still hear so much about the dangers of cholesterol? Avoiding cholesterol is not critical, taking vitamin E is!

Just a few words now about "eggs." The egg has been sorely maligned. In studies done by Dr. Roger Williams, eggs were the one single food that can sustain life indefinitely on a monodiet. To omit them from one's diet would be a tragic mistake. Noting now how relatively unimportant dietary cholesterol is, it has nonetheless been shown that the intake of cholesterol, especially from eggs has little to do with increasing one's total serum cholesterol. Although there are only two references cited here, there are many others that confirm the statement that "egg consumption does not affect serum cholesterol levels." 14.15

Now we shift our attention to the real problem, the problem that has been causing nearly half of the total deaths in the United States. That problem is the inadvertent development of blood clots in our circulating blood. One generalized term for this is "thrombogenesis." A thromboembolus can be any foreign body in the blood circulatory system. This can be the dislodging of a piece plaque from an artery or a vein, or the formation of a clot by the process that we know as "platelet aggregation."

From what I describe above, you now understand that in certain conditions plaque can develop within the circulatory vessels. It can occur in either the arteries or the veins. Sometimes, perhaps caused by a blow or trauma to a limb, a piece of plaque can be dislodged. This can occur sometimes for no apparent reason. If for example this happens in a vein of the leg, the particle of plaque will travel with the blood flow to the heart and then to the lungs where it can become lodged. Wherever the particle lodges, the tissues on the other side of the blockage will be starved of nutrients and oxygen. This is called an "infarct." If the circulation to an infarct is not immediately resumed, those tissues will die. This can happen in any part of the circulatory tree, arteries or veins as the vessel branches become smaller and smaller.

Another more common occurrence is platelet aggregation. I mention above that platelets carry within them chemicals that cause them to aggregate or clot. This has a very important purpose, which is to prevent excessive bleeding when injury occurs. The problem with platelet aggregation is that it can sometimes occur too readily. The reason is that people are eating the wrong type of food ‾ more specifically, the wrong type of fat, including both liquid oils and solid fats.

Two words that are very important in understanding these concepts are "thromboxane" and "prostacyclin." Thromboxane is found within the platelets and is released during their fracture, and consequently is an important defense against excess bleeding during injury. As platelets fracture or are exposed to the air, they form clots to stop the flow of blood. This substance is abbreviated as TXA2.

In opposition to the clotting action of thromboxane is another chemical called prostacyclin. It is the job of prostacyclin to dissolve blood clots and to dilate the blood vessels. This is abbreviated as PGI2.

These two chemicals are supposed to work in harmony so that clotting occurs only with injury, but does not occur within the blood vessels. The main nutritional sources for these chemicals are various fats (oils) from the diet. The problem arises when these two chemicals, thromboxane and prostacycline, are produced from common vegetable oils, causing the TXA2 to be much too clotty, and the PGI2 to be not potent enough to dissolve the internal clots and to dilate the blood vessels. The result is a body chemistry that too easily forms blood clots by platelet aggregation.

In our chapter on Vitamins, Minerals and Food Supplements, we discuss the very unique situation that science has found among the Greenland Eskimo population. In brief, it has been discovered that the Greenland Eskimo has the lowest coronary heart disease rate in the world, even though their diet consists of 70 percent of their calories as fat. This seemed unbelievable until it was understood that the fat they consume is considerably different than what we eat.

This is the reason: in order to prevent fish from solidifying in the extremely cold water of the Arctic, nature provides a very unique type of oil. Originating in the bodies of tiny plankton, which are eaten by the krill, and then eaten by larger fish and seals, this very special oil moves up the food chain to the Eskimo. Once within their bodies, this oil has a profound effect on the human production of very different thromboxane and prostacyclin. It produces a thromboxane that is not very clotty, and a prostacyclin that is very anti-clotty. These are abbreviated as TXA3 and PGI3 respectively. These are very different from the thromboxane and prostacyclin produced in oils from temperate climates, and, hence, the reason why there is such a low incidence of coronary heart disease among the Greenland Eskimo. And, this is the reason that this unique oil is a beneficial addition to anyone's diet. 16, 17, 18, 19, 20, 21.22

The oil from the cold-water fish is termed "Omega III" oil, and within it are some very important fatty acids not found in temperate climate oils. These are eicosapentaenoic acid (EPA) and docosahexaenoic acid (DHA). Don't be confused by these names, but become acquainted with these letters.

The shortage of Omega III essential fatty acids could be the most critical deficiency in the American diet. The question that presents itself is, can these fatty acids be obtained by eating fish several times each week? The answer is, only if the fish has been living in frigid water, and only if it had the opportunity to eat the tiny plankton that produce this wonderful oil. Simply increasing your fish intake does not guarantee that you are getting sufficient EPA and DHA. However, there are a number of companies that harvest the oil from fish in the extremely cold Arctic waters in the winter and early spring when the EPA and DHA content is at its highest. This is encapsulated and can be taken as a food supplement, and I recommend it highly as a measured source for this wonderful nutrient.

Another condition called "variant angina" should be discussed at this point. Part of the makeup of a blood vessel is the muscular wall. Variant angina is a condition that occurs when the muscles of the walls of the blood vessels go into spasm. I can remember reading an article many years ago published in one of the newsmagazines. It described a team of Italian surgeons in the midst of a coronary bypass surgery. They remarked that at a certain point, the coronary vessels visibly went into spasm. They described it as though "someone was wringing them out." This offers an explanation as to why some surgeons who might diagnose atherosclerotic blockage in a patient by symptoms and surgically go in to remove it, find nothing since the spasm may last only several seconds or minutes!

What happens in variant angina is simply the spasm of an artery. Many times it is of only short duration, but gives the exact symptoms of angina pectoris. In what we call "differential diagnosis," the difference between angina pectoris and variant angina can sometimes be determined by the time of its occurrence. If it occurs during heavy exercise, it would more than likely be angina pectoris, a blockage by plaque. If it occurs during rest, it would more than likely be variant angina. 23, 24, 25.26

But, the good news is this: the prostacyclin produced from fish oil as described above has a profound effect on relaxing the muscles of the arterial walls! So, the miracle of Omega III fish oil serves not only to prevent platelet aggregation, but also to prevent the vasospasm of variant angina.

You have heard that it is a good idea to reduce the fat in your diet. This is sound advice. Above I have described the dangers of trans fatty acids from hydrogenated oil, but there is something to be said about natural fat as well. I refer to research done by George Miller, a researcher at St. Bartholomew's Hospital in London. He found that even one high fat meal could bring on a heart-damaging clot. In a report that he gave to an American Heart Association's annual science writers meeting in January 1993, he stated that a high fat meal can trigger rise in a certain "factor VII" which is a protein that triggers a cascade of blood clotting events. In other words, a fatty meal late in the evening can trigger a heart attack in the early hours of the morning when this factor VII is at its highest. 27

Now let's talk about strokes. A stroke is indeed a type of vascular disease. But instead of affecting the heart, it affects the circulation within the brain. There are three types of strokes:

The first is caused by a blood clot in the arteries to or within the brain.

The second is caused by a blood vessel bursting in the brain.

The third is caused by vasospasm similar to variant angina described above.

As mentioned above, a blood clot can occur anywhere within the arterial or venous blood vessels. If it occurs in the vessels of the heart, it causes coronary occlusion. If it occurs in a lung, it is called a pulmonary occlusion. If it occurs in the brain it is called a stroke. 28 Each type of stroke should be differentiated because an episode will require different diagnosis and treatment. If the type of stroke is caused by a blood clot, then the prevention is exactly as mentioned above for platelet aggregation. Vitamin E and the Omega III fats would be extremely important. However if the stroke were the second type, caused by a burst blood vessel, the treatment and prevention would be entirely different, perhaps even requiring surgery.

In the case of an occurrence of a burst blood vessel in the brain, two factors are extremely important. The first of these is the status of collagen in the body. Collagen is connective tissue, the glue that actually holds the cells together. This reticulum or collagen also holds the cells of the blood vessels together. In the disease called scurvy, caused by a severe vitamin C deficiency, one of the symptoms is hemorrhage in various tissues, easily seen as red blotches under the skin. 29 This should be a great indicator of a connective tissue problem, but sometimes it is not so apparent, because there can be a breakdown of the tissues of the blood vessel walls without being evidenced in the outer skin. Connective tissue is nourished by not only vitamin C but also by the flavonoids and bioflavonoids found in many fresh fruits and vegetables.

The second critical factor in this type of stroke is increased blood pressure. The chances for a burst blood vessel in the brain are greatly increased if there is a deficit of vitamin C. When under the stress of increased blood pressure, it is possible that the weak areas in the connective tissue of the artery might give way. If this happens within the brain, a stroke occurs. When this happens, and depending on the size of the breach, blood leaks out of the artery into the tissue spaces, forming a hematoma, which is a pool of blood within the tissue spaces. The hematoma takes up space within the brain, causing pressure on the surrounding brain tissue. The size of the hematoma will determine the neurological symptoms caused by it. Sometimes the hematoma is small and will cause minimal neurological damage, but sometimes it is large and can severely *damage that person's brain to the point of causing paralysis or death.*

With regard to these two types of stroke, an accurate diagnosis by the attending doctor is absolutely critical. Let me give you an example. Let us assume that an individual is having a hemorrhagic stroke. A vessel within the brain has ruptured. Immediately a clot begins to form to stem the internal blood flow.

If the stroke is caused by a clot, immediate treatment by a physician with one of the new "clot busting" drugs can actually minimize the brain damage by breaking up the clot before the brain cells are irreparably damaged. The danger occurs with a misdiagnosis. If a hemorrhagic stroke is treated with clot busting drugs as the ruptured vessel is attempting to stem the blood flow with a clot, the clot will be dissolved and the bleed will continue. The ensuing hematoma could be fatal.

The last type of stroke is caused by vasospasm, which is a spasm within a blood vessel in the brain (variant angina). With this type of stroke, damage is usually minimal, and recovery can be complete within several weeks. Once again, prevention of this type of occurrence would be the use of the Omega III oils which effect the relaxation of these arterial muscles via the production of PGI3.

Summary – Cardiovascular disease is disease of the heart or blood vessels. It can affect the heart as atherosclerosis caused by plaque; it can be a clot caused by platelet aggregation; or it can be variant angina caused by a spasm of the muscular walls of a blood vessel.

A stroke can be a burst blood vessel within the brain, a blood clot within the brain, or a variant angina caused by spasm of one of the blood vessels leading to or within the brain.

There are numerous nutritional factors that can increase or reduce your chances for cardiovascular disease. Let me list them for you here.

Factors that increase your risk of cardiovascular disease:
a high fat diet
rancid fats
"trans" fatty acids
constipation
ionizing radiation (which can be received from X-rays or even high altitude flights)
chlorinated water
homocysteine

Factors that reduce your risk of cardiovascular disease:
B complex vitamins especially B6, niacin, and riboflavin
vitamins A, C, and E

minerals including zinc, manganese, selenium, molybdenum, copper, magnesium, and chromium.

cysteine, an amino acid available in eggs and other complete protein sources

beta carotene

garlic

fiber

yogurt

beans

alfalfa seeds and sprouts

vegetables

cold-water fish and Omega III oils

exercise

lycopene, one of the carotenoids found in tomatoes

monounsaturated fats (olive oil)

heparin (released during fasting)

tocotrienols (part of the vitamin E complex)

CARDIOVASCULAR REFERENCES

1. http://library.louisville.edu/government/goodsources/deaths.html

2. Enos WF, Holmes RH, Beyer J. Coronary disease among United States soldiers killed in action in Korea: preliminary report. JAMA. 1953; 152: 1090–1093.

3. McNamara JJ, Molot MA, Stremple JF, et al. Coronary artery disease in combat casualties in Vietnam. JAMA. 1971; 216: 1185–1187

4. http://carlisle-www.army.mil/apfri/chapter_3.htm

5. http://www.hsph.harvard.edu/reviews/transfats.html

6. http://www.americanheart.org/presenter.jhtml?identifier=180

7. http://heartdisease.about.com/cs/cholesterol/a/raiseHDL.htm

8. http://www.mercola.com/2003/jul/19/trans_fat.htm

9. U.S. News and World Report. May 31, 1993. p. 80.

10. Esterbauer H. Dieber-Rotheneder M. Striegl G. et al; Role

of vitamin E in preventing the oxidation of LDL. *Am.J. Clin. Nutr.* 1991: 53: 314S-321S.

11. Kok F. van Poppel G. Melse J. et al. *Atherscler* 1991;86:85 – 90.

12. Dieber – Rotheneder M, Puhl H, Waeg G et al. J Lipid Res. 1991;32;1325 – 1332.

13. *American Journal of Clinical Nutrition.* January 1991.

14. Edington J. et al. Effects of dietary cholesterol on plasma cholesterol concentrations in subjects following reduced fat, high fiber diet. Br Med J. 1987; 294:333.

15. Flynn M, Nolph G. Osio Y, et al Serum lipids and eggs. J Am Diet Assoc. 1986; 86: 1541- 1545.

16. http://www.ajcn.org/cgi/content/full/74/4/415

17. http://www.ajcn.org/cgi/content/full/ajcn;74/4/464

18. www.issfal.org.uk/Abstracts-Wed.

19. Trapani FJ; Health Discovery of the Century. WCA Journal. 1984

20. Trapani FJ; Eicosapentaenoic Acid and Thromboembolic Disease. ACA Journal; April, 1986.

21. Sanders TAB. Dietary Fat and Platelet Function. Clinical Science(1983) 65, 343 – 350.

22. Eskimo Diets and Diseases. The Lancet. May, 21. 1983.

23. http://www.americanheart.org/presenter. jhtml?identifier=4472 - 40k - Apr 15, 2004

24. http://www.sbrmc.com/html_healthgate/html/0_453/45390. php - 42k

25. www.escardio.org/knowledge/cardiology_practice/ ejournal_ vol2/Vol2_no9.htm - 44k - Apr 16, 2004 –

26. www.sh.lsuhsc.edu/fammed/OutpatientManual/Angina. htm

27. U.S. News and World Report. Feb 1 1993 p.69.

28. Nutritional Data. International Research Center. April 1960. pp45,46.

29. Kutsky, R.J.Handbook of Vitamins, Minerals and Hormones. Second Edition. 1981 Litton Publishing Co. p.257.

8.

CANCER

Abstract

*E*ven though cancer is the second leading cause of death in our culture and as yet know little about cancer mechanisms we can still overcome this disease. With the help of studies this chapter will guide you through the list of factors that encourage cancer as well as those that prevent it. You will find that there are considerably more anti- carcinogens than there are carcinogens. Our task is to teach you to balance these factors towards the preventive side, and there are considerable nutritional factors that can do just that!

Of all the topics we cover in this book, cancer is the most difficult to explain. The reason is because there are more than 200 types identified with many instigating causes. Cancer is the second cause of death in our country after cardiovascular disease.

In this chapter my goal is to answer your question "is there anything I can do to reduce my chances of getting cancer?" In my opinion, there is.

Let's begin with some background.

Here are some of the factors that are involved:
Your diet
Your immune system (which indeed is closely connected with your diet)

Your age
Your genetic make up
Viruses.
Your environment

There are three words that we should define before we begin:

1. **Carcinogen** – A cancer causing substance.

2. **Mutagen** – Any agent including radioactive elements ultraviolet radiation and certain chemicals that causes biological mutation (the altering or changing of the cell).

3. **Teratogen** – An agent that induces abnormalities in a developing embryo or fetus.

<u>Your diet</u> – For my way of thinking this topic leads the list. Even though the "experts" state that diet is probably responsible for only 1/3 of the cancers, I believe from experience, research and reason that the figure will eventually be found to be closer to 2/3. The reason is because of the importance of the immune system in preventing cancer, and because of the importance of diet in maintaining and strengthening the immune system.

Whenever we discuss diet we invariably must mention not only the positive and negative things that we eat, *but also those things that we don't eat*. Things for example, that our immune system needs to remain effective and to do its job properly.

I have put this chapter last because after reading to this point, you will have a good idea of what your diet should include and those things that you must avoid.

At the end of this chapter I have a list of the carcinogens and anti carcinogens that you should become familiar with.

When speaking of diet and the chemicals in our environment the first thing that the skeptics will bring up is that cancer has been around long before man-made chemicals. Yes, we do know and must agree that although there are many carcinogens in our environment, and although they have been around for thousands of years, there are many more man made carcinogens now as well.

For example rancid fats, aflatoxins on certain grains and peanuts, burnt fat, and moldy foods have been around as long as man. But we must also agree that man has come up with many as well. These would be synthetic food colors, preservatives, synthetic hormones etc. But just as there are carcinogens in our diets and surroundings, there are also numerous anticarcinogens that can protect us!

When reading the lists below I believe that you will come to the same conclusion as I, that if we can outweigh the carcinogens with more anticarcinogens and if we indeed keep our immune systems healthy , we might greatly improve our chances to avoid this disease.

Your immune system – Because of its importance, we have devoted an entire chapter to the immune system. As I mention there, it is the immune system that protects us from things within the body as well as things outside the body that would harm us.

For example if a body cell starts to mutate into a cancer cell, a healthy immune system will automatically destroy it before it can grow into a tumor. So, as important as it is to protect us from exposure to bacteria and viruses, it is equally important to constantly maintain a healthy immune system to protect us from cancer. The immune system will function properly only if all of the necessary nutrients are present. If only one vital nutrient is missing, this system may not function properly and hence rid the body of those damaged cells. This may be speculation, but I believe it to be founded on reason.

Genetics – Within each cell of the body is found the nucleus of that cell. Within the nucleus are found tiny bodies called chromosomes and within them are many genes. These genes hold the blueprints for the production of other similar cells. These genes can be altered by exogenous or endogenous (from outside or from within the body) chemicals and factors. Some of these genes have been identified as having a predisposition towards cancer. But contrary to what you might think, even if a person has identifiable genetic predisposition, this does not insure that that person will get cancer. Many individuals who have genetic predisposition do not get cancer. This can only mean that there are still other factors that must be brought into the equation to produce cancer.

Your age – As I mention above, there has to be a number of changes occurring to the genes within a cell before it turns into a cancer cell. In most cases, some carcinogen has damaged the cell. There is also the possibility that the damage occurred when that cell was formed. In either case, the damage is passed on to the daughter cells when those cells divide. It stands to reason that the longer we live, the more time there is for us to accumulate these genetic mistakes in our cells. Yet, once again as I mention above, it is the job of the immune system to rout out and destroy these cells before they begin their process of multiplication into a tumor. So, even in these cases, a healthy immune system is vital.

Viruses – Apparently certain viruses can be the cause of specific cancers. In such cases, the virus causes the genetic changes within the cell that makes it more likely to become cancerous. I must comment again that an intact immune system should remove these imperfect cells before they begin to multiply into tumors.

Some examples would be cervical cancer caused by the genital warts virus and liver cancer caused by the Hepatitis B virus.

The environment – Where a person lives and works can be the determining factor for the risk of cancer. We can name any number of factors within this category that could contribute to the development of cancer. There are too many to list here, and I'm sure you can come up with an endless list. But just to name a few the list would include:

Over exposure to the sun.
First hand and second hand cigarette smoke
Natural and man-made radiation
Many types of smoke and fumes
Radon naturally occurring in soil
The list could be extensive. 1

Dietary Factors that can cause cancer

Increased fat intake – (the term 'fat' includes oil as well as solid fat) Numerous studies indicate that the more fat in the diet, the greater chances are for certain types of cancer. Once again the type of fat must be taken into consideration. The most dangerous fat would be the man-saturated fat that contains trans-fatty acids. Most of the studies seem to indicate that saturated fat increases the risk of colon cancer. This seems to prove the point that food such as those containing a great deal of fat will slow down peristalsis (the intestinal movements that push the food through the digestive tract). This will cause fecal matter to remain in the colon longer with greater risk of developing carcinogens from bile and other chemicals present. Combining vegetables in meals with their fiber will encourage greater peristalsis and reduce this possibility.2, 3,4.

Rancid and Peroxidized and Heated fat – Fat can become rancid inside as well as outside of the body. Statistics indicate that fat accounts for around 40% of the U.S. diet. One of the greater problems with fat is its ability to become rancid. When this happens it causes a chain reaction to occur producing a variety of mutagens and carcinogens.5

It is also suspected that over consumption of vegetable oils might promote certain types of cancer. 6.

One of the greatest dangers with fat is the matter of overheating it. Pan frying, Deep fat frying (French-frying) and Barbecuing all cause the fat to molecularly break down. Not only does this produce trans-fats, but other mutagens and carcinogens as well. It would be well to note that the accepted visual sign of this occurrence is when the oil or fat begins to smoke. Whether pan-frying, French-frying or barbecuing the fat is usually brought to this temperature very quickly. With each of these events, you can be assured that the fat has been damaged and may be dangerous.8.9.

Mold and aflatoxins – Mold that can sometimes be found on food such as peanuts, peanut butter, other nuts can contain a serious carcinogen called aflatoxins. In actuality, it is said to be one of the most potent carcinogens. 5

Tobacco products – If enough hasn't been said about the carcinogenicity of tobacco, we will add another flame to the fire by stating that there is also sufficient evidence to prove that there is an increased cancer risk in adulthood from early life exposure to parents smoking.7.

Burnt Protein and caramelized sugar – Almost any overheated protein food or sugar that is heated to the browning point may contain mutagenic material. In a comparison of the amount of mutagens and carcinogens taken in by two pack a day smokers as compared with the amount taken in from burned or browned foods, Americans in general seem to get more carcinogens from the browned food, especially barbecued meat 5.

Mushrooms – Most common mushrooms contain substances called hydrazines. Almost all hydrazines are known to be potent mutagens and carcinogens. These are found in most mushrooms including the widely used false morel (Gyrometra esculenta) as well as the most common commercial mushroom (Agaricus bisporus).5.

Nitrates and nitrites – Those people that derive their drinking water from wells in agricultural areas should have their water tested for nitrates and nitrites on a regular basis. These chemicals are used in agricultural fertilizers and can leach down into the ground water, and into wells. The other source for these chemicals are from all preserved meat. Hot dogs, pepperoni, salami, bologna and virtually all sandwich meat will contain these chemicals. As we mention in our chapter on Food Additives, nitrates and nitrites in themselves they are marginally carcinogenic, but if and when they combine with amines (protein breakdown products) in the stomach, they can form some of the deadliest carcinogens known, called nitrosamines. 5.

Potato glycoalkaloids – If you have ever grown potatoes in a garden, you will have noticed that if they are not hoed to mound the soil around the plant, some potatoes will be exposed to the sun. When they are, they develop a green color. Within that color is found some very potent teratogens. These can also develop if the potato is bruised or diseased. The substances formed are called chaconine and solanine, and in heavy doses can be lethal to humans. As an example, more than 40 mg. of glycoalkaloids in a 200 gm potato is considered to be a toxic level. It should be noted if you carefully examine your potatoes and detect this green color, it can be cut off and the rest of the potato is safe to eat.5.

Food additives and pesticides – It is difficult to say which food additives might be carcinogenic, and there are more than 5,000 found in our foods. You can find some answers in our chapter on this subject.

Cottonseed oil - There is a major toxin in cottonseed oil called gossypol. This substance is recognized as being a carcinogen as well as a mutagen. When a list of ingredients on a food label states "vegetable oil" as one of its ingredients, more than likely it is cottonseed oil. Besides containing gossipol, there is a strong chance that it may contain various pesticides and other farm chemicals. The reason for this is that cotton has virtually no restrictions on what may be used in its growing. Hence, the seed may very well contain many of these chemicals. Cottonseed oil is probably the cheapest oil on the market. 5.

Perhaps it is best to say here that with this information we should not become discouraged nor paranoid about the food we eat.

Yes, these factors are around us, but typically occasional exposure to any of these is not significant. It is the frequent, continual exposure that makes the difference.

For example, I am reminded of a man in one of my nutrition classes many years ago.

We were discussing the carcinogenicity of burnt protein and heated fat. A man in his mid thirties raised his hand and said "what you are saying is quite true". He continued by saying that he was single, lived alone, had a good job, and cooked at home. His favorite meal was steak. But he described that he liked his steak cooked in a very special way. He would heat a fry pan, put the steak into it, and burn it quickly dark on each side, and leave the steak quite rare inside. He commented that the steak would sizzle and the smoke would rise from the burning fat. And that was how he prepared his steak! So, I asked, what's your point? "Well", he said, "last year they found cancer and had to remove about half of my stomach".

You see, it's not the occasional exposure to the carcinogen, but its continual use.

If, for another example, you like French fries and hamburgers, bearing in mind that the oil in the French fryer at the local hamburger joint may be filtered, but is seldom changed. You can be assured that it has reached the smoking, carcinogenic stage many times. Eating fries occasionally will probably have little effect, but eating them many days each week may indeed irritate the stomach lining to the point of affecting the cells and initiating a cancer.

Factors that can prevent cancer.

The cruciferous vegetables – This includes cabbage, broccoli, brussels sprouts, cauliflower, kale and possibly watercress and bok choy. Apparently the cancer protection factors involve the presence of thousands of phytochemicals that have anticancer properties. Some of these are glucosinolates, crambene, sulforaphane and indole-3-carbinol (I3C) which specifically changes the way estrogen is metabolized, and hence may prevent estrogen driven cancers such as breast cancer and perhaps many other types of cancer as well. 10.11. Now recognized as forms of nutrients, these isothiocyanates are found only in the cruciferous vegetables. But even more exciting is the fact **that broccoli sprouts contain 20 to 50 times more sulforaphane than you find in mature broccoli.** To extrapolate those figures, it means **that you will get as much sulforaphane from a few tablespoons of these sprouts as you would in a pound of broccoli.**

Watercress contains a powerful compound called phenethyl isothiocyanate (PEITC) which is not only a general cancer preventive, but also specifically blocks the nicotine in cigarette smoke from causing lung cancer in animals.12,13,14.

I feel very strongly that the more cruciferous vegetables in your diet, the less your chances are of getting cancer.

<u>The carotenoids</u> – Surely, we have all heard of beta carotene. It is but one of the miracle nutrients that we find in many vegetables and certain other foods such as eggs. But few people know that beta carotene is only one of perhaps 500 – 600 other carotenoids found in nature. Of those that have been studied, science has thusfar isolated *beta carotene, lycopene and canthaxanthin, lutein, zeaxanthine, and cryptoxanthine*. Their action seems to be due to their wonderful antioxidative capabilities.

Hundreds of studies have been published concerning their anti carcinogenic capabilities.

A recent study was done at the Division of Gynecologic Oncology at the Albert Einstein College of Medicine in the Bronx, N.Y. Within a cross sectional sample of 235 women, it was found that those with cervical cancer had a significantly lower blood plasma level of canthaxanthine, lycopene and beta carotene. 15.

In other studies, lycopene, which is found in high concentrations in tomatoes, had a profound effect on preventing prostate cancer as well as cancers of the bladder, cervix, colon, rectum and skin. 16. These results were incurred with 4 to 10 servings of tomatoes each week.

According to Dr. Graham Colditz of Harvard University older Americans "who often ate tomatoes in abundance were only half as likely to die from all cancers combined". 17

Apparently lycopene is not destroyed by cooking and hence is available from a multitude of products besides fresh tomatoes.

As a point of importance, beta-carotene has been synthetically made. Some of the studies that were done with this synthetic substance have had less than desirable results. Once again I reiterate, stick with naturally occurring nutrients.

There are literally hundreds of studies in scientific literature confirming the anti cancerous effect of many nutrients. I list below some of these that I hope will convince you of the importance of nutrition concerning this disease

Once again in keeping with my comments in our chapter on vitamins, minerals and food supplements, I strongly urge the use of only natural nutrients as well as natural carotenoids. My recommendations will always state that the natural sources are the best. But for a concentrated natural source of all of the carotenoids, there can be nothing more potent than carrot juice.

Additional sources for your information are listed in our references for this chapter:18 – 40.

HERE IS A QUICK REFERENCE OF MANY CARCINOGENS AND ANTICARCINOGENS

CARCINOGENS

HIGH FAT INTAKE	NITRATES
OXIDIZED FATS	ALCOHOL
TRANS FATTY ACIDS	POLYUNSATURATED OILS(OVERUSE)
IONIZING RADIATION	LOW SERUM CHOLESTEROL
AFLATOXINS	CAFFEIC ACID (IN COFFEE)
CIGARETTES	REFINED CARBOHYDRATES
BURNT FAT OR PROTEIN	OBESITY
CERTAIN MUSHROOMS	POTATO GLYCOALKALOIDS
CARAMELIZED SUGAR	MANY FOOD ADDITIVES
EXCESS IRON	MANY PESTICIDES
COTTONSEED OIL (GOSSYPOL)	SOME DRUGS
MOULDY FOOD	

ANTICARCINOGENS

ANTIOXIDANTS; (CAROTENOIDS; VITAMINS C,E; SELENIUM; CO Q 10; FLAVONOIDS

LOW FAT DIET

SELENIUM

VITAMIN C

CRUCIFEROUS VEGETABLES

THE CAROTENOIDS

THE B COMPLEX VITAMINS

VITAMINS A; D; K;

CALCIUM

EXERCISE

ZINC

OMEGA III FISH OILS

HIGH FIBER DIET

GARLIC

UNREFINED CHO'S

MANGANESE

MAGNESIUM

MOLYBDENUM

LOW CALORIE DIET

CANCER REFERENCES

1. http://www.cancerhelp.org.uk/help/default.asp?page=90

2. Hursting S, Thornquist M, Henderson M: Types of dietary fat and the incidence of cancer at five sites. Prev. Med 1990; 19: 242-253.

3. Whittemore A, Wu-Williams A, Lee M, et al: Diet, Physical activity and colorectal cancer among Chinese in N. America and China. J Nat Canc 1990;82:915-926.

4. Giovanniucci E, Stampfer M, Colditz G, et al: Relations of diet to risk of colorectal adenoma in men. Am J Epidem 1990;132:783

5. Bruce N. Ames, Dietary carcinogens and anticarcinogens. Science; 23 Sept. 1983. Vol. 221; 1256-1264.

6. Fernandez G, Inhibition of pulmonary metastasis of B16 melanoma variants by saturated dietary fat intake. Clin Res.1986;34:A562.

7. Sandler D, Everson R, Wilcox A,Browder J; Cancer risk in adulthood from early life exposure to parents smoking. AJPH May 1985, Vol. 75, No. 5

8. V Archer; Diet, Cooking Methods, and Cancer. Health Media of America, The Nutrition Report; Vol. 6 No 12; Dec. 1988.

9. Steineck G, Hagman U, GerhardssonM et al Vitamin A supplements, fried foods, fat and urothelial cancer Int J Canc.1990;45:1006-1011.

10. http://www.healthcentral.com/DrDean/DeanFullTextTopics.cfm?ID=11172

11.http://www.lef.org/magazine/mag2000/july2000_i3c.html

12. http://www.nih.gov/news/pr/sep2000/niehs-18.htm

13.http://www.aicr.org/information/foods/cruciferous.lasso

14.http://www.femalemuscle.com/nutrition/cruc_veg.html

15.http://www.ncbi.nlm.nih.gov/entrez/query.fcgi?cmd=Retrieve&db=PubMed&list_uids=9816105&dopt=Abstract

16. http://www.leffingwell.com/lycopene.htm

17.http://www.tribuneindia.com/1999/99mar10/health.htm

18. Knekt P, AromaaA, Maatela J,et al: "Serum vitamin A and subsequent risk of cancer" Am J. Epidem 1990 :132: 857 – 870.

19. Barbone F, Austin H,Austin J,et al: Diet and endometrial cancer. Am J Epidem 1990;132:783.

20. Hsing A, McLoughlin J., Schuman L, et al. Diet, tobacco use and fatal prostate cancer. Cancer res. 1990; 50:6836-6840.

21. Heilbrun L, Nomura A, Stemmermann G: Black tea consumption and cancer risk.Br J cancer1986;54:677-683

22. Colacchio T, Memoli V: Chemoprevention of colorectal neoplasms. Arch Surg 1986;121:1421-1424.

23. Hann H, Blumberg B: (high)Iron nutrition and tumor growth. P Am Assoc Ca 1987; 28:158

24. Schatzkin A, Jones D, Hoover R, et al Moderate alcohol

consumption and breast cancer. N Eng J Med 1987; 316: 1169-1173.

25. Heimberger D, Alexander CBirch R., et al Folic sacid and B 12 beneficial in treatment and prevention of lung cancer. Am J Clin Nut 1987;45: 866

26. Hsing A Comstock G, Abbey H,et al: Vitamin A and prostate cancer linked. J Nat Canc 1990: 82; 911-916.

27. Giovanucci E, Stampfer M, Colditz G, et al. High saturated fat, low fruit, vegetable intake linked to colorectal cancer. Am J Epid 1990; 132:783.

28. Victor Archer MD. Diet, Cooking Methods and Cancer. The Nutrition Report Vol 6 No. 12 Dec 1988.

29. Van T, Veer P, Kolb C, Verhoef P, et al. Breast cancer risk reduced by fiber, increased by dietary fat. Int J Canc 1990; 4: 825-828.

30. Steineck G, Hagman U,Gerhardsson M et al; Fried food affects uninary cancer risk. Int J Canc 1990; 45: 1006-1011.

31. Robert L, Stalder R, Dombrowsky I, et al: Low calorie diet reduces cancer risk.Int J Vit Nutr Res 1985: 55: 452.

32. Brock K, Mock P, Berry G, Beta carotene reduces risk for cervical cancer. Am J Epidem 1986; 124: 518.

33. Cameron E, Bland J. Balance of omega 3 and omega 6 oils and their relationship to cancer.Nut Res vol 9 1989.

34. http://www.ars.usda.gov/research/publications/Publications.htm?seq_no_115=153970 Effect of cruciferous vegetables in preventing cancer.

35. Arbman G, Axelson O, Ericsson-Begodzki A, Fredricksson M, et al. Mineral deficiencies associated with increased incidence of colorectal cancer. Cancer 1992;69: 2042-2048.

36. Comstock G, Bush T, Helzlsouer K, Low intake of antioxidant nutrients linked to cancer risk.Am J Epidem 1992; 135: 115-121.

37. Lin X, Liu J, Milner J: Garlic powder an effective anti cancer agent. FASEB J 1992; 6: A 1392.

38. Paganelli G, Biasco G, Brandi G, et al: Vitamins A,C and E prevent cancer.

39. Weinzweig J, Mendecki J, Friedenthal E, et al. Vitamin A and Argenine shown effective in cancer treatment. Fed Proc 1986:45: 1078.

40. Szeluga D, Bistrian B, Mascioli E. Fish oil prolongs life, slows tumor growth. Am J Clin N 1987; 45: 859.

9.

MEAT AND POULTRY

Abstract

*R*ecently with the fear of Mad Cow Disease ever present on our minds, most people are unaware of the fact that this is only the tip of the iceberg concerning the chemicalization of our meat supply. In this chapter we discuss the many chemicals, hormones, antibiotics and diseases that are present in our beef and poultry that most of us consume every day. After reading this chapter you may feel the need to become a vegetarian. Although as yet I haven't gone that route, and still feel that meat can be an important one's diet, I can confess that the meat my family eats is carefully chosen.

The controversy about meat is ongoing. Should it be part of one's diet? Can we deny the fact that many cultures have existed on meat as the prime source of protein for many generations? So, with the ethical aspect aside, just how good is meat as human food? What does it provide in our diets?

Nutritionally, meat ranks in the top three categories with eggs and fish as the best sources of complete protein (containing all eight of the essential amino acids). Meat also has a very high NPU (net protein utilization) factor, which means that a good amount of what is eaten is actually utilized by the body. Therefore, if there are no ethical concerns, if it is "good meat", and if it is consumed in moderation, it can be an important part of our diet.

As with other food, when we talk about meat, we must understand that the main problems associated with meat are in its production. It is essential to learn how our meat is raised, how it has been processed, exactly what has been added to it, and also how it has been cooked.

Let's discuss some of the controversial topics about meat:

The chemicals

Preserved meats such as hot dogs, sausage, jerky, ham, bacon, salami, pepperoni, and bologna all contain chemicals, principally sodium nitrate and sodium nitrite, in order to preserve the color and to protect from contamination by bacteria. But do these chemicals cause harm to our bodies?

As mentioned earlier in the chapter on food additives, we can have short-term reactions, long-term reactions, and chemical interactions. Even if we agree that the nitrites are only marginally harmful in small amounts, in the arena of chemical interactions, we find a more sinister problem. In the acidic environment of the stomach, sodium nitrite may combine with amines (the breakdown products of protein) to form a chemical substance called "nitrosamines." Some scientists are greatly concerned because nitrosamines are some of the most potent systemic carcinogens, (meaning that they can cause cancer in any part of the body). In other words, even if we accept the argument that nitrates in small amounts are harmless (which I find hard to believe) then the fact that they interact with the amines in your stomach is certainly a good reason to exclude them from your diet. A better alternative is to use fresh meat ⁻ just cook it at home and slice it for sandwiches. It is an extra effort compared to just picking up the luncheon meats in the grocery store, but by taking the extra time, you'll be getting your protein with fewer additives. 1, 2, 3

Hormones

Some years ago the pharmaceutical industry succeeded in creating a synthetic copy of an important female hormone. This hormone called "stilbesterol" was synthesized in the laboratory, **but the final product *was not the exact duplication of the original*.** The resultant synthetic hormone was called *"diethylstilbestrol."* Although it seemed to duplicate most of the needs of stilbesterol in the body, its side effects were monumental.

One of the two arenas where diethylstilbestrol was problematic was in human pregnancy. In the complex cycle of pregnancy, there is a prime hormonal change at the end of the first trimester. At that time the natural hormone stilbesterol should start to be released. If it is not perfectly coordinated with the diminishing of other hormones, the mother will start to abort. The first sign will be that she will start bleeding vaginally. It was found that if these women were given the synthetic hormone diethylstilbestrol, the pregnancy would be sustained. This was a great achievement for the medical/pharmaceutical industry. As it turned out however, this synthetic drug is a deadly carcinogen, and as those children whose mothers were given this synthetic hormone reached puberty, a certain percentage of the females developed cervical cancer while the male offspring developed testicular cancer. 4

At first, the reports claimed that only one in 10,000 would have the problem; new statistics however indicate that the figure may be closer to one in 25 or fewer!! I have personally spoken with a number of those individuals who told me that they are encouraged to go for medical checkups on a regular basis. My niece happens to be one of those unfortunate women who developed cervical cancer from this synthetic hormone.

But that's only half of the story. It became apparent at the onset that this same synthetic hormone could be used in another way. The agricultural industry is always interested in ways to increase what they call "the grain-to-gain-ratio" which, in other words, is how a grower can get more meat with less feeding of grain. Along these lines, the pharmaceutical industry sold the farmers the idea that if they used this hormone, they would need less grain to fatten their animals. At first, a capsule filled with this hormone was implanted in the tissues under the skin of the neck of the animals. It released this hormone like a gland over the growing period of the animal until slaughter, causing a change in the sexual hormonal balances. After several years of use, it became apparent that certain problems were arising. Of prime importance was the fact that the tissue around the implant contained an inordinate amount of the hormone, and if eaten could cause cancer. Secondly, it was found that male individuals who inadvertently consumed more of this hormone were showing signs of "gynecomastia," a condition of enlarged breasts in men. 5, 6, 7

After about five years of use, when these side effects were confirmed, the practice of neck implants was discontinued. The use of this hormone in farm animals was abandoned for several years until the pharmaceutical industry found that they could make it in the form of a powder and put it into the livestock feed. This practice continued for many years until there was enough of an outcry concerning its carcinogenesis (cancer causing effects) that that practice was also discontinued. But it was not stopped until there were other products in the wings ready to take over. 8

This is the scenario thus far: A synthetic sex hormone, used to prevent spontaneous abortions in women, caused cancer in a percentage of the male and female offspring of the recipient. This same synthetic hormone was used to increase the grain-to-gain-ratio in farm animals. Although the agricultural industry knew via the Delaney Amendment that it was allowed a zero tolerance of this chemical in meat, *traces were found in carcasses and reported by several whistle-blower inspectors* 9,

10 (The Delaney Amendment, passed in 1958 forbade the use of any additive that might cause cancer.)

Now, here is the kicker. The medical community now knows that an embryo in the first weeks of life in the womb can be influenced and affected by an infinitesimally small amount of any harmful chemical. In fact, the figures quoted state **that an embryo can be affected by 1/10,000 the amount that would affect an adult.** So the fear has been, and still is, that the reason for the current high number of cases of cervical cancer in women and testicular cancer in men is because their **mothers ate meat tainted with the synthetic hormone diethylstilbestrol at the critical stages of their pregnancies.** 11

The question we must now raise is whether the newer hormones being used currently have inherent dangers that have not yet come to our attention.

Here are some of the products that are now being used in our farm animals (to the best of my knowledge, all are administered via ear implants) ‾ Zeralanol; Synovex; Cattlyst; Revalor S; Rumensin; Component TH; Monensin and Finaplix.

Zeralanol is an anabolic agent that stimulates the pituitary gland to produce increased amounts of somatotropin, a hormone that promotes growth.

Synovex has been modified by the addition of trenbolone acetate, which is an androgen-like compound. Several of the products contain estrogen and estrogen-like compounds as well as progesterone compounds. **Cattlyst** contains a recently approved substance called laidlomycin propionate, a drug from the category of chemicals called collectively ionophores.

Very interesting to me is a warning presented on a label of one of these products which states, **"Do not attempt salvage of implanted site for human or animal food."** Many countries around the world forbid the use of these drugs and chemicals in their meat production ‾ do they know something that we don't know? Are they being wisely cautious while we are not? 12,13,14,15

Antibiotics in meat

It has been speculated that pathogenic antibiotic-resistant organisms are being created because of the overuse of antibiotics prescribed by physicians. That is only half of the truth. The other part is the use of antibiotics in farm animals.

Any time bacteria are exposed to an antibiotic, they are under what is called "selective pressure" which allows only resistant forms to survive and reproduce. So the basic rule to curtail this evolution of resistance must be to reduce unnecessary use of antibiotics.

Antibiotics have been used in our meat supply for two basic reasons. First, and less problematic, is that antibiotics are routinely used when farm animals become sick. Farmers in this country are allowed to treat their own stock, which they do on a regular basis. If an animal looks sick, or goes off feed, a farmer may decide to put the animal on an antibiotic regimen.

The grower may in some cases decide to take the animal to the stockyards for slaughter immediately while it is still on the antibiotic regimen, rather than taking a chance of losing the animal altogether. The problem here is that there is frequently a residual antibiotic presence at the site of injections, usually in the rump, where some of the best cuts of meat are taken. If a person who consumes the meat from that site is allergic to that particular drug, there may be an allergic reaction. In some cases, this may be a severe reaction that will not likely be connected to the antibiotic residue in the meat.

But a far worse problem has arisen with another use of antibiotics in our meat. Approximately 40-45 years ago, once again, in an attempt to increase the grain-to-gain ratio in farm animals, the farmers were told that by including some powdered antibiotics in with the feed their animals would gain weight faster and cheaper. Farmers began utilizing antibiotics in the livestock feed at that time, and as a matter of fact are still doing so. According to studies done in the 1960s, there was considerable controversy as to whether or not antibiotics even worked for this purpose. Let me reiterate that the livestock were fed antibiotics not to control disease, but rather to increase the grain-to-gain ratio. 12

In the first week of June 1967, The National Academy of Science and the Food and Drug Administration (FDA) held a public symposium in Washington D.C. on "The Use of Drugs in Animal Feeds." Then commissioner Dr. James L. Goddard presented the many years of scientific concern with antibiotics in animal feed. He stated that this practice is a dangerous one because it offered the possibility of bacteria mutating and becoming dangerous in several ways. First that they might become insensitive and resistant to antibiotics, and also that they might mutate and become pathogenic and excessively dangerous to mankind.

It has taken more than 40 years, but that which was feared has come upon us. You no doubt have heard of *salmonella, e coli, listeria* and a number of other drug-resistant pathological organisms that we now must deal with. Antibiotic-resistant bacteria may transfer resistance genes to other bacteria, via so-called horizontal gene transfer, and these resistant bacteria can then be transferred between animals and between animals and people. 16,17,18

Now comes the interesting part of the story. An outbreak of an intestinal disease occurred several years ago in the United States caused many restaurants to close and many people to get sick and indeed for some to die. Yet the full story was never disclosed by the major news media. You may recall some of the outbreaks of *salmonella* and *e coli* diseases that occurred in certain restaurants. Unfortunately, in most cases, the main responsibility for these problems was incorrectly laid to rest on those specific restaurants. Indeed, some of the blame did rest on them for not cooking the meat thoroughly. But you must understand that the bacterial contamination was already in the meat when they received it. Not only was the meat already tainted with bacteria, it was tainted with these "super-bugs" that were not only resistant to antibiotics but highly pathogenic as well. What I am saying is that those truly responsible for this problem were never exposed.

In one of these cases, some wonderful detective work was done by the Centers for Disease Control. The contaminated meat was traced to a single farm in the Midwest where the inevitable had happened. The continuous use of antibiotics in the feed to increase the grain-to-gain ratio caused a mutant variety of *salmonella* to be generated. It was not only pathogenic, but it was resistant to antibiotics. Many individuals who ate this meat became severely sick with intestinal disease. The big problem arose however when in an attempt to control the disease they were given oral antibiotics. The result was that several individuals died. 19

Understand the twist here. When the individual ate the contaminated meat, and the organisms infested their intestinal tract, these organisms had to compete with the normal intestinal bacteria, which in most cases offered competition to the growth and multiplication of the mutant organisms. But when oral antibiotics were introduced for the intestinal distress caused by eating the bad meat, or for any subsequent malady, all of the normal, friendly bacteria were killed off, leaving the resistant pathogenic organisms to flourish, free of competition. In the cases of *e coli*, byproducts called *Shiga* toxins were secreted which caused tremendous damage to the human host, including acute hemorrhagic colitis (painful, bloody diarrhea), hemolytic uremic syndrome (HUS), as well as another condition called thrombotic thrombocytopenic purpura (TTP) . Similar cases were reported all around the country including in our small town of Walla Walla, Washington. In total, here in Walla Walla, 34 cases were reported to be caused by the lethal bacteria *e coli* 0157H7 resulting in several deaths. In these cases, "inspection of the restaurants disclosed no sanitary violations or unsafe practices." 20 Of course, the problem was already present in the meat!

Although some of the blame for spreading this disease rests on poor sanitation in the processing plants and the restaurants, and also in the undercooking of meat in the restaurants, the true culprits, in my opinion, are the pharmaceutical companies and the agricultural industry for introducing and continuing the use of antibiotics as a feed additive. 21

A recent study by the Union of Concerned Scientists revealed that **every year in the United States, 25 million pounds of antibiotics are fed to livestock as a feed supplement.** This drug load represents a full 70 percent of the total U.S. antibiotic production. Human medicine, in comparison, uses only 3 million pounds of antibiotics each year. 23

Fast food hamburgers
Did you know that there is a "claim to fame" in the fast food hamburger industry? Truthfully, I don't believe that it matters much as far as quality is concerned, but it is an interesting story anyway. The United States Department of Agriculture (USDA) grades beef into eight specific categories: prime, choice, select, US standard, commercial, utility, cutter, and canner. These grades reflect primarily the amount of marbling or fat within the muscle fibers, and hence, the tenderness of the cuts. Almost all of the cuts of meat used as steaks and roasts are of the first four grades. The lower four are rather tough, grading down to canner, which is the toughest. In other words, you cannot use commercial grade beef or below as steak. It's just too tough.

When living and practicing in Hawaii some years ago, I had several radio programs in which I did health exposés and commentaries for many years. One such exposé concerned this topic of meat. After the broadcast, the manager of one of the biggest meat packing plants in the Islands contacted me. He invited me to inspect their plant in order to show me the quality of their meat. During that meeting and review of the facilities, he conceded to me that indeed, hamburger is made from the lower grades. His comment was that although the meat is tougher, once it is ground into hamburger, it really doesn't matter. Furthermore, he said that the tougher grades, which frequently come from old milk cows and old bulls really made a tastier hamburger. This makes good sense to me because it would make a more flavorful hamburger, as is the nature of meat from older animals.

But here's the kicker. Fast food hamburger franchises use these cheaper, **leaner** grades of meat. They are allowed 30 percent fat by law in their hamburgers. Since the cheaper grades of beef are relatively lean, **the franchiser makes up the difference by *adding cheap fat* from processing plants up to the 30 percent limit**. This is the trick to the financial success of most of the fast food hamburger joints!

POULTRY

Chickens and turkeys are graded by USDA standards. For the most part, the grading is related basically to the appearance of the carcass, including whether or not there are any visible cuts, bruises or broken bones. In other words, it seems that the standards have nothing to do with the quality of the meat or to tenderness, but simply its appearance. Furthermore, *the grading and inspection process is a totally voluntary one* for which the producers must pay to have USDA graders. *Large processing plants have their own inspectors who are trained and approved by the USDA. So, in essence, the producers are actually grading their chickens themselves ⁻ a literal example of the fox guarding the henhouse!*

Most commercial poultry are raised in large flocks, sometimes numbering 20,000 to 100,000 birds. This is usually done in large sheds on a concrete floor covered with shavings. 21 For the most part, the type of chicken sold for eating falls into two general categories: fryers and broilers. With that basic understanding, the interesting facts are these: broilers and fryers raised in such large numbers and in severely crowded conditions are fed antibiotics from day one to control disease, and also to speed up the growth with less feed. 25

I maintain that the use of antibiotics in chickens presents exactly the same problems that it does in beef.

Broilers are usually slaughtered at 7-8 weeks, and fryers from 4-7 weeks. In other words, these are young chickens and consequently the most tender.

Stewing hens are typically old laying hens. Being older they are much tougher and hence must be stewed, or cooked for a long time. These are considered the tastier chickens for soup; hence when you buy prepared chicken soup, it is usually from stewing hens. But, I see no particular problem with that.

With that in mind, I might just comment here that shark and bovine cartilage has been touted as being excellent for health in several ways, both as a cancer preventative and cure, and also excellent for joint health. But let's not forget the time-honored cure for colds and flu and just about everything else: chicken soup. I suspect that chicken soup does have curative aspects that no doubt come from the dissolving of some of the chicken cartilage in the soup made from the long-stewed chickens.

Diseased Animals

Well, if what you have read thus far doesn't make you a more careful meat shopper, or indeed a vegetarian, then this might. Recently, I have learned that the USDA has passed some new regulations that allow the sale of meat from animals and poultry that have tumors, pus, sores and scabs. 26 Yes! And the reason stated for this allowance is that these animal diseases are not transmitted to humans....yet! I add the word "yet" because haven't we learned a lesson from the fact that the AIDS virus did jump from animals to man? And even more recently that the monkeypox virus did the same?

Nevertheless, even if this is only a matter of repugnance, do you want to eat that kind of meat or poultry? I first read about this problem in a report published in *"Restaurant News"* in 1970, entitled "USDA May Give O.K. to Tumored Chicken." The concern was that the virus involved in causing disease, called the "leukosis virus" or *Myeloid Leukosis* (ML), might cause leukemia in humans. This proved at that time not to be true. However, the immediate problem for the growers was **that the disease caused *repugnant-looking skin lesions*. According to the report, the panel of government scientists recommended that the tumors or lesions could be "cut out" and the *remainder of the bird sold as "cut-up chicken."*** And further, the recommendation went on to say that ***"the tumorous portion could be ground into hot dogs."*** 27 Researcher Michael Worsham writes, "Poultry plants often salvage meat, cutting away visibly diseased or contaminated sections, and selling the rest as packaged wings, legs or breasts, according to 70 inspectors." Richard Simmons, an inspector at a ConAgra plant said, "Practically every bird now, no matter how bad, is salvaged. This meat is not wholesome. I would not want to eat it. **I would never, in my wildest dreams, buy cut-up parts at a store today.**" 28 and all this while you thought that the chicken was cut up as a convenience to you? If there is any question about the veracity and accuracy of these data, I suggest that you research my references.

A more recent development is the arrival of an even more serious poultry disease called Avian Leukosis Virus (ALV-J) that can cause all sorts of ills in poultry, including respiratory disease, tumors of the bones, liver, spleen and kidneys, and increased mortality. So serious is this disease that *it is threatening virtually all breeding flocks in the United States.* 29, 30

Regarding the bacterial contamination of poultry carcasses, it was reported by Reuters news service on Tuesday, December 10, 2002, that the Consumers Union said the previous week that it analyzed 484 raw chickens purchased at supermarkets in two dozen U.S. cities. Of these chickens, **42 percent were contaminated with *campylobacter* and 12 percent with *salmonella*.** 31

The Humane Society of the United States reported early in 2004 about disease causing bacteria present in our poultry. In October 2002, Pilgrim's Pride recalled 27.4 million pounds of chicken because the meat was suspected to be contaminated with the organism called *listeria* which was implicated in much illness and several deaths in humans in the northeastern U.S. 32

MAD COW DISEASE (BSE, or CJD, & vCJD)

Mad cow disease is the newest threat to those who consume meat, as well as to many others. Although it is recognized as being a neurodegenerative disease, there is still much that is unknown about it ⁻ but what we do know is very frightening.

The disease is not new, and has been recognized for over 300 years as "scrapie," a disease of sheep and goats in the British Isles. Two scientists are credited with the first descriptions of the disease as early as the 1920s. The scientists whose name it carries were Creutzfeldt and Jakob, hence the name Creutzfeldt-Jakob Disease, (CJD). After additional study of this disorder, other researchers determined that the condition called "kuru" found in the Fore people in the highlands region of Papua New

Guinea was the same or similar disease to CJD. That area is the first known to claim the disease in humans. Its transmission there was believed to result from the consumption of brains during cannibalistic funeral rituals.

As an affliction of animals, the vast majority of mad cow disease incidents have occurred in the United Kingdom where more than 180,000 cases have been reported since 1986. In humans as CJD, the disease has been around for many decades, affecting about one person per million due to genetic or other unknown causes, and affecting mostly those within the range of 50–75 years of age.

After the kuru episodes detected in New Guinea, it again began appearing in humans elsewhere in the world. The first reported case involved a 19-year old man in the United Kingdom in 1994. Whereas CJD affects mostly the elderly, the new variety known as "variant CJD" (vCJD) seems to affect younger people. Furthermore, there is little doubt that eating infected meat transmits the disease.

One of the most curious differences with this disease is that in animals the incubation period is 3-8 years, and in humans the incubation period is at least 5 years and possibly longer than 20 years! With no known cure, the gruesome disease begins with mood swings, numbness in various parts of the body and uncontrolled body movements. Eventually, Alzheimer-like memory problems become apparent as the disease spreads too much of the brain tissue, finally resulting in death. Autopsy of such individuals reveals much of the brain as literally eaten away and looking sponge-like, hence the name bovine spongiform encephalopathy, (BSE).

The disease is believed to be caused by tiny particles called "prions" which are a form of protein found in the nerve cells of all mammals. In theory, a person ingests meat or another animal product containing abnormally shaped prions. The prions then get absorbed into the blood stream and cross into the nerve tissue. The abnormal prion touches a normal prion and changes the normal prion's shape into an abnormal one, thereby destroying the normal prion's original function. These abnormal prions continue contacting and changing other normal prions. The nerve cell then tries to get rid of these abnormal prions by clumping them together in small sacs called lysosomes within the affected cells where they accumulate. As the lysosomes become engorged within each nerve cell, that cell eventually dies. When that cell dies it bursts and releases the abnormal prions within, which then infect other cells. The final outcome is the formation of large sponge-like holes where many cells have died.

But the question that begs an answer is, "why now?" If the only other recorded human outbreaks of this disease were in New Guinea, and they were caused by eating human tissue, what is causing it now? The scientific consensus is that the feeding of animal by-products to other animals sets up a dangerous possibility of the disease. In that manner, the abnormal prions are transferred from the feed containing infected animal tissue to the next animal within its feed. It is then transferred to humans who consume that animal.

The most audacious aspect of the matter is the same agricultural mentality that says "do anything to make the bottom line better!" As mentioned above, feeding hormones and antibiotics to increase the grain-to-gain ratio is a common practice, but the growers have taken it a step further by feeding rendered animal parts to animals that are and always have been vegetarians!

Since 1989, bovine spongiform encephalopathy (BSE) has been identified in twenty European countries, Japan, Israel and Canada, with one uncertain case within the U.S., which was believed to have been brought in from Canada.

There are several other disturbing facts. The question still remains whether these prions can be carried in any animal product other than food. It should be understood that gelatin capsules and other gelatin products, drugs, vaccines, tissues such as would be used in transplants, and cosmetics all contain animal products. We do not have the answers, and due to an incubation period that could stretch out to two or more decades, we may not have an answer until the problem is pandemic!

While the FDA has supposedly stopped the importation of animal products from countries that have documented cases of BSE, it is possible that some could still be getting through. Drugs and vaccines including those given to millions of American children have been made with products that could potentially have carried mad cow disease. Nine different vaccines, which have been given to millions of Americans, include polio, diphtheria and tetanus. They also include the anthrax vaccine that has been given to virtually all soldiers serving in the Persian Gulf Region. 33, 34, 35, 36, 37, 38, 39

RECOMMENDATIONS

In light of the above, what course of action should we take regarding poultry? I still feel, as do many nutritionists, that meat can be an important part of our diet. It is a high quality and highly concentrated complete protein. By that I mean that it contains the eight essential amino acids necessary for human health. But it must be clean, wholesome, and free from drugs and other hormones and chemicals, and from feed that contains animal byproducts.

I would venture a guess and say that unless you are living in some remote part of the country, that there is almost assuredly someplace near you where you can purchase "organically grown" meat and poultry. Search it out! If you live in an agricultural area as my family and I do, then find a farmer or rancher in your vicinity that will produce such meat for you and your friends.

And, for that matter, offer a higher price for the meat. It will be well worth it for you. Furthermore, tell your friends and family what you have learned here and encourage them to buy organic meat, both for their own health and also to support the organic farmer.

Regarding the tenderness of meat, it is not absolutely essential that the meat you buy be of the higher grades. Indeed, prime and choice grades are the most tender, but they also contain the marbling, which provides the most undesirable fat. If you are fortunate enough to have access to a farmer who grows clean drug-free meat, he will more than likely know that even grass fed beef can be reasonably tender. The trick is that they must be slaughtered while they are "on the gain" or putting on weight quickly while on pasture alone.

I can guarantee that as more people become conscious of these facts and demand cleaner, disease-free and drug-free meat, the larger companies will take notice and begin to provide it. We still live in what is known as a "market society", and the market for good meat will ultimately decide what quality of meat is available to us.

References; Meat and Poultry

1. " Effect of Frying and other Cooking Conditions on Nitrosopyrrolidine Formation in Bacon" J.W. Pensabene, et al. University of Minnesota Extension Bulletin. FS-00974. http://www.extension.umn.edu/distribution/nutrition/DJ0974.html.
2. S.R. Tannenbaum and T.Y. Fan in "Uncertainties about Nitrosamine Formation in and from Foods," proceedings from the Meat Industry Research Conference, University of Chicago, 1973,
3. W. Fiddler, et al. (J. Food Sci., 39:1070, 1974)
4. Wall Street Journal – Aug 3, 1972
5.http://www.emedicine.com/plastic/byname/gynecomastia.htm

6. http://www.emedicine.com/med/topic934.htm

7. http://www.transadvocate.org/des51.htm

8. HEW News 72-70 Aug 7, 1972

9. Washington Post Service; October 17, 1971

10. National Health Federation Bulletin; January 1970

11. Medicine Today – Ladies Home Journal; November. 1971

12. http://www.ralgrocanada.com/en/starteng.html

13. http://www.ansi.okstate.edu/research/2000rr/09.htm

14. http://www.extension.iastate.edu/Pages/ansci/beefreports/asl-1452.pdf

15. http://www.lambriarvet.com/catalog/cattleimplants.htm

16. http://whyfiles.org/038badbugs/scope.html

17. http://www.ems.org/antibiotics/antibiotics_food.html

18. http://www.northstar.sierraclub.org/antibiotics/factoryfarms.asp

19. Washington Post; September 6, 1984.

20. Walla Walla Union Bulletin; Dec.3, 1986.

21. Letters to the Editor; Townsend Letter for Doctors. Dr. F.J. Trapani p. 235

22. http://scienceweek.com/1998/sw980220.htm #15

23. Additional references;. Refer to Google search engine: "Antibiotics in Meat"(115,000 references shown). "Antibiotic Use in Farm Animals" 35,801 references shown.

24. http://www.vegsoc.org/info/broiler.html

25. http://www.hsus.org/ace/14485

26. http://www.organicconsumers.org/toxic/chixpus.cfm

27. Washington Report: Restaurant News. February 16, 1970.

28. http://www.rtis.com/reg/bcs/pol/touchstone/September95/health.htm

29. http://www.ars.usda.gov/is/AR/archive/aug98/viru0898.htm

30. http://www.ag-web.com/agissues/aii9981102/alvj02.html

31. http://www.organicconsumers.org/irrad/poultrybacteria.cfm

32. http://www.hsus.org/ace/14485

33 http://www.mad-cow.org/

34 http://www.fda.gov/oc/opacom/hottopics/bse.html

35 http://www.cdc.gov/ncidod/diseases/cjd/cjd.htm

36 http://www.organicconsumers.org/madcow.
37 http://whyfiles.org/012mad_cow/
38 http://science.howstuffworks.com/mad-cow-disease.htm
39 http://www.cjd.ed.ac.uk/

MILK AND DAIRY PRODUCTS

Abstract

*M*ilk and its products have always been and always will be a staple in our diets.

But as with many of our other food staples, dairy foods have undergone some damaging changes. How valuable is dairy in our diets? Is all milk the same?

Is it necessary to pasteurize? Is raw milk safe? Are chemicals or hormones added to the milk? What about other dairy products such as cheese and yogurt are they valuable and safe? In this chapter we discuss these subjects.

Milk and other dairy products have long been the subject of a great deal of discussion within the field of nutrition, from the accusation that cow's milk is the ideal food "only for calves", to the statement that milk is one of the few complete foods for humans. Which is correct?

In my contacts and study for the past 40 years, I personally have met with many of the people making many of the above statements. Some of the "experts" will not touch milk because it causes "mucus." Others will not touch milk because it's an animal product, others because has too many chemicals and hormones. What is the truth? Let's discuss it.

One of the most important papers I have ever read on this subject was published in 1971 by a man who I believe stands out in clinical research, Roger J. Williams. The paper is entitled "The Nutritive Value of Single Foods." 1

This study began out of one particular experiment that Dr. Williams did wherein he found that when he fed normal enriched white bread to them, weanling rats died within several weeks. His experiments were criticized by some of his colleagues who felt that white bread is never eaten alone, but always with other foods. More specifically, his colleagues remarked, "The experiments that you performed would have given the same or similar results if you had begun with milk, meat, eggs or any other food."

Dr. Williams' skepticism about this statement encouraged him to go ahead and test these single foods to see if indeed the results would be the same. The following foods were tested by being given singly to groups of twelve animals: pasteurized vitamin D whole milk; hamburger meat cooked twenty minutes; all-meat commercial precooked frankfurters; fresh eggs steamed ten minutes; canned tuna; roasted peanuts; shredded wheat breakfast cereal; wheat flakes breakfast cereal (commercially enriched); puffed rice, (commercially enriched); and macaroni (commercially enriched). **The results showed *that eggs, by far, succeeded in sustaining life indefinitely*.** Second only to eggs was milk, but only if supplemented with iron and copper. Third on the list was hamburger, but not close to the excellent results obtained with eggs. All of the other test items were what I would call "dim failures," unable to sustain life. But even though milk was second on the list, it is fully capable of sustaining life with the addition of those two minerals. To me this puts milk into a rather esteemed position along with eggs ‾ certainly a food that should be utilized.

Let's start with some of the procedures concerned with milk production.

Diet

Whether talking about human milk, cows' milk or goats' milk, *the quality of the milk is directly related to the diet of the mother.* All human milk is not necessarily the same nutritionally. 2 For the same reasons, all cows' milk is not the same nutritionally. Certain nutrients such as the minerals calcium, phosphorus, and magnesium, as well as protein, and many of the vitamins can have a direct effect on the quantity of the milk produced, and hence, on the offspring being fed it. But many of the trace minerals such as selenium, zinc, manganese and many others can be deficient or missing entirely with little effect on the quantity of milk produced. In the same manner, researchers have recently determined that the Omega III fatty acids EPA and DHA as well as arachidonic acid are extremely important for the development of the brain in newborn infants. If they are absent in the mother's diet, they will likely not be present in her milk. 3

Hence, a cow should have a high protein diet, sufficient roughage, access to pasture and quality feed, and some multi-mineral supplement. In addition, a quality farm will feed extra, natural vitamin supplements.

Pasteurization

Just what is pasteurization, and what is it for? Let's start from the beginning. Going back a few years, milk was produced by a multitude of small farms. Some consisted of large herds and some of smaller herds. Each farm could not bottle and sell its own milk. That is an entirely different business. Hence, dairies were established with bottling facilities. These dairies bought the milk from each individual farm, and bottled it under a corporate name. In the "old days" it was common to see many 5-gallon milk containers from the morning's milking on the country road waiting for the dairy pick-up each morning. Let me stress at this point that milk is an excellent medium for the production of bacteria. They thrive on it! They breed in it!

Let's assume that Farmer #1 on the dairy pick-up route is a conscientiously clean individual. His barn, his animals, his containers are always meticulously cleaned and sterilized. Farmer #2 on the route however has only a few animals but sells his milk to the same dairy. He's too busy to tend to the few cows, so he assigns the chore to "Junior" who doesn't bother to wash his hands after shoveling the manure, and then milks the cows by hand. He also fails to wash out the buckets and milks into yesterday's pails (which are never washed out either.) Do you get the picture? This is a breeding ground for some very bad bacteria.

When the milk from these two or more farms arrives at the bottling dairy, it is all mixed together, the clean with the dirty. Milk produced in an unclean manner can be downright dangerous! So over time, the dairies adopted the practice of running all the milk through the pasteurizer.

Most people don't quite have the correct picture as to just what the pasteurization process does. Pasteurization *does_not* sterilize the milk! It simply reduces the total bacterial count. Another misconception is that pasteurization destroys only the bad bacteria. Again, not so! Pasteurization brings down the total count of both good and bad bacteria to the level that humans won't get sick from it. To accomplish this, the milk is heated to 63 °C (145 – 150 ° F) for not less than 30 minutes (slow pasteurization) or to 72 ° C (163 ° F) for not less than 16 seconds (flash pasteurization). Recently a newer form of pasteurization is being used that indeed does sterilize the milk. This is called UHT pasteurization (ultra high temperature) and it is accomplished at 141 ° C, or 285 ° F for one to two seconds. 4 In essence, this process entirely sterilizes the milk so that no bacteria, neither good nor bad, remain. Milk sterilized with this method can be made to stand unspoiled for many days, even at room temperature, as long as the carton is unopened. The disadvantage is that vitamins, mostly the B vitamins are "heat labile." meaning that they are unstable and can be destroyed by excessive heat. 5, 6

Each form of pasteurization takes its toll on the nutritional quality of the milk, either in the destruction of vitamins, amino acids, and enzymes. This process is being used extensively in the dairy industry, and I believe that someone should do an assay to determine just how much nutritional destruction occurs with each type of pasteurization. Before I go on, let me reiterate once more that raw milk can be dangerous! But it does not have to be.

Raw Milk

Now let's go back to our story about the two dairy farmers. We understand that raw milk can be dangerous ‾ but it does not have to be! What if each dairy were absolutely scrupulous with cleanliness? Would the milk still require the nutritionally destructive pasteurization? The answer to that question comes from a multitude of "raw milk dairies." Let me tell you about one that I knew very well. It was called the Walker-Gordon Dairy in Plainsboro, New Jersey. Although they are no longer in existence, I can speak from personally having been there. They milked about 1,750 cows. The cows received no hormones of any kind. They were fed a highly nutritious diet of quality hay, grain, and silage with special supplements like brewer's grains, malt sprouts, linseed meal, soybean meal, bran, and molasses In other words, their nutritional intake was exceptional. As I mention above, from a nutritious diet comes exceptionally nutritious milk..

These well-nourished cows were milked twice a day with an ingenious invention called the "rotolactor." This was a sort of a large merry-go-round fitted with stalls around the periphery. The cows were led up to the rotolactor, and before entering, each received a shower and was wiped down with sterile towels. A special attendant then washed the udders with a disinfecting solution. The cow then was made to step into a rotolactor stall where another attendant fitted the disinfected milking machine, beginning the milking process. The fresh milk was delivered directly up into a glass container where the quantity was measured and recorded. It was then piped directly into the milk bottles. In other words, the milk was never exposed to the air. At the end of the cycle of the rotolactor, the forward gate was opened and the cow walked forward off the machine and back to her stall. The wonderful fact was that the bacteria count of the raw milk from this dairy was lower than the bacteria count of the pasteurized milk from other dairies! *Now, that is the way that milk should be produced!* Furthermore, each cow was inspected and tested by veterinarians on a regular basis for any and all diseases. If a cow showed any signs of a problem, she was immediately taken out of production.

Although I am not familiar with any of the certified raw milk dairies currently in existence around the country, let me say that I'm sure that the milk from those dairies must be regularly inspected. 7, 8 Once again, we must understand that the quality of milk is directly related to the methods of production and diet. For the most part, dairy animals must be fed reasonably good diets in order to sustain their milk production. But there are some mineral nutrients that do not affect the volume of milk produced. If a cow is deficient in those minerals_ it still can produce quantities of milk, but the milk will not contain the deficient minerals. For that reason you would want to find a dairy that produces milk from quality feed, preferably from an inspected and certified raw milk dairy.

Dairy hormones
Now, let's get to an even more serious problem, the problem of hormones. Virtually all commercial dairies (except those designated "organic") are using hormones to increase milk production. In other words, fewer cows, more milk! Among these hormones are the following:

BGH (Bovine Growth Hormone)
rBGH (recombinant Bovine Growth Hormone)
bST (Bovine somatotropin)
rBST (recombinant Bovine somatotropin)

These products are used to increase a cow's milk production. The recombinant varieties are genetically engineered, and the cows are needle injected with these hormones every 2 weeks. To make this synthetic product, some tissue is snipped from a cow with DNA that codes for this hormone. This is inserted into the DNA of *E coli* bacteria (found in all feces) which is grown in vats, yielding large quantities of rBGH. **Many countries including Norway, Sweden, Denmark, the Netherlands and the Canadian Provinces of Alberta, British Columbia and Ontario have banned commercial use of these hormones. What do they know that we don't know or are willing to admit?**

One of the lesser problems from the use of these hormones is the increase of udder infections (clinical mastitis.) These are then treated with antibiotics, which of course find their way into the milk. According to the General Accounting Office (GAO), the FDA has approved of 330 antibiotics on dairy cows, and an additional 50 antibiotics are suspected of being used illegally. In addition to the mastitis, these products are associated with an increase in bovine cystic ovaries, increased digestive disorders such as indigestion, bloat and diarrhea.

Monsanto, the company that introduced these products into the market, has succeeded in convincing the FDA that other dairies may not label their milk "free of hormones." 9 They have convinced the FDA that there is no difference between the milk of treated and non-treated cows, and they maintain that a label saying "rBGH free" would imply a difference that does not exist. Monsanto has filed lawsuits against milk processors who label their product "free of rBGH"!

Some independent studies have already suggested that there is a distinct possibility that the rBGH may lead to allergic reactions in consumers.10

Another factor of great concern in hormone produced milk is that it causes an increase in an insulin-like growth factor (IGF-1.) Although milk ordinarily contains this factor, and although it is necessary for human growth, researchers have found up to 10 times the amount in milk from cows treated with these hormones. The question remains, what effect does this increased amount have on the human body?

The concern is that because this substance is a growth-promoting factor that it will increase the growth of cancer in humans, especially prostate cancer in men, and breast cancer in women. 11,12,13,14,15,16,17

Like most chemicals, hormones and other additives to our food, this is yet another factor that we must worry about. Like so many cases in the past, the true harm of these substances is not totally revealed until many years later. I consider this to be human experimentation, and we are the guinea pigs! Many assurances from the FDA and industry-paid consultants do not convince me of its safety. We know now that Bovine Growth Hormone (BGH) in its many forms is banned in Australia, New Zealand, and Japan. Also, the European Union has maintained a moratorium on milk products from rBGH and BST treated cows, and such products are not sold in countries within that union. Even Canada has thus far resisted the pressure from the biotechnology lobby to approve the commercial use of rBGH. Are we so absolutely sure that our science is so much clearer than theirs?

Homogenization
Most of you who are reading this now probably don't remember the days long ago when it was necessary to shake a bottle of milk before using it! Milk fat or cream, being lighter

than the milk itself, would rise to the top of the container. Mom would even steal a bit of it for her coffee before shaking the bottle. Nowadays, separation does not occur, due to homogenization, which is a process whereby the fat particles of the cream are reduced in size so that they remain dispersed indefinitely. Is this good or bad?

In research done by Dr. Kurt Oster, MD, he cites that the reduction in size of the fat globules in the cream also reduces the size of a substance within the cream called "xanthine oxidase." This substance in itself would not pass through the intestinal membrane unless thus reduced in size. In the homogenized state, it can pass through and may indeed be a major factor in atherosclerotic disease. Other research from NASA finds that increased XO may also have a profound effect on the eventual cause of lipid peroxidation (you might call this the beginning of rancidity of the fat), membrane damage, and even cell death. 18,19

So, once again we are left to determine if indeed this process to our food is damaging to our health. Unless you have a source of clean, inspected raw milk, you are left to choose whether or not to consume homogenized, pasteurized, and ultra-pasteurized milk.

Dairy Products

<u>Natural cheese</u> ‾ In general, most cheeses are made from pasteurized cow's milk, although some are made from the milk of other animals such as goats and sheep. In the production of cheese, the factors within the milk are separated into curd and whey. This is done by the action of rennin (an enzyme) or special bacteria. These products can then be further divided into two very broad categories – fresh and ripened. The fresh cheeses are cottage cheese, pot cheese, ricotta, and cream cheese. In order to become ripened cheese, the curds must be "cured" by a variety of processes such as heating and addition

of various bacteria . The curds may also be flavored with salt, herbs and other spices. This product is then allowed to ripen and age during a controlled storage period. There are many unique methods used to obtain different flavors and textures in the final product.

Processed cheese – Here we start running into certain procedures that become questionable to me. The production of processed cheese may begin with a natural cheese, but it is then pasteurized to lengthen its shelf life. It may have emulsifiers added to it to aid smoothness. Some processed cheeses contain coloring agents and preservatives. Products labeled "cheese spreads" and "cheese foods" may contain added liquids to create a more spreadable product. *Government standards allow such products if only 51 percent of the product is cheese.*

Fermented dairy products
Fermented dairy products can be divided into three classes :
1.   *Liquid products which include acidophilus milk, buttermilk, kefir and koumiss*
2.   *semi solid products which include cultured cream and yogurt*
3.   *unripened soft cheeses, which include cottage cheese, and cream cheese.*
Of all of these, I personally feel that yogurt, kefir and acidophilus milk are the most important ones, hence the ones we will discuss.

These products contain very special bacteria that convert the milk sugar lactose into a mild acid called "lactic acid." Aside from those special bacteria, additional bacteria are used in these products for flavor. Because of the special ecology within our digestive tracts, these lactic acid bacteria are very helpful in maintaining certain chemical balances. You very well could call them the "good bacteria." The acidity that they produce is helpful in maintaining the proper acid/base balance within the intestines, and their acid secretions discourage the growth of many of the harmful bacteria. It also is believed to enhance digestion and improve the absorption of nutrients into the body. A few of the more prevalent bacteria used in fermented dairy products includes

L.Bulgaricus,S.Thermophilus,L.acidophilus,and*bifidobacteria*. Collectively, the study and practice of maintaining these good bacteria is called **"Probiotics."**

Although the history of fermented milk products dates back perhaps thousands of years, we can say with fairly good certainty that the original purpose for making yogurt was to preserve milk. Prior to the modern innovation of refrigeration, there had to be some way to prevent milk from spoiling. If a cow on a single family farm gave more milk than that family could consume within one or two days, the milk simply soured, due to the multitude of bacteria in the environment. Since milk is an excellent culturing medium, all types of bacteria that got into the milk including airborne bacteria, fungal spores and yeast. These survived and thrived, making the milk sour.

<u>Yogurt</u> – (*streptococcus thermophilus* and *Lactobacillus bulgaricus*)

To make yogurt, the milk must be sterilized. beyond the capability of pasteurization. That means that all contaminating bacteria, fungal spores and yeast must be destroyed. This is done by bringing the milk temperature to the "scalding" point, which is the temperature just before the milk boils. This must be done in order to prevent the culturing of undesirable and dangerous organisms. The milk is then cooled down to just the right temperature and the new desired culture of bacteria is introduced. The temperature must then be held at a specific temperature for several hours for these good bacteria to multiply within the entire batch. As I mentioned above the very fact that they secrete a mild acid is the reason why the yogurt will stay longer before spoiling. 20, 21

Studies have recently shown that the long-term daily consumption of 300 grams of yogurt over a period of 21 weeks increased the serum concentration of HDL cholesterol (the good cholesterol) and led to the desired improvement of the LDL/HDL cholesterol ratio. 22

You will note that one of the bacteria mentioned above is *L. Bulgaricus*. It was thus named because modern yogurt was originally taken from Bulgaria. Even though yogurt supposedly goes back thousands of years, this is where modern yogurt was originally found. Let me draw you a picture of the process used to make yogurt in Bulgaria for hundreds of years. Most homes had fireplaces for heating and cooking. Each fireplace had a swinging "arm" onto which could be hung an iron cauldron. The extra milk was put into that cauldron and swung into the fire. It was kept there until just before boiling. The cauldron was then swung somewhat away, but still near enough to keep it warm. When the lady of the home decided it was the correct temperature (108 - 112 degrees F) 24, she introduced some yogurt from a previous batch, and then swung the cauldron to just the right place that would keep the exact correct temperature. There was one extra "trick" that was used to make a superior "thicker" yogurt. If the milk was kept at the scalding stage for many hours, not boiling, but just right, much of the water of the milk was driven off, leaving a higher concentration of milk solids. This made a thicker more desirable yogurt.

Kefir – (Kefir grains *Streptococci spp*, *Lactobacillus caucasicus*, *Leuconostoc spp*., and yeasts)

Kefir is another important lactic acid product.. In contrast to yogurt, which contains good, but "transient" bacteria, the bacteria in kefir will form colonies (called grains) which attach to the intestinal walls. In other words, yogurt must be continually eaten to maintain a population within the intestines, kefir forms colonies that are attached to the walls of the intestines which will continue their good work for longer periods of time. The proper culturing temperature for kefir is also different, being about 64 -75 degrees F. Although some authorities maintain that it originated in northern Africa, there is much consensus that its origin is from the Caucasus mountain area of the east. 25 In any event, the drink was originally fermented naturally in bags made of animal pouches. The "grains" attached themselves to the walls of these pouches, and the person needed only to refill the bag with new milk and wait about 24 hours to enjoy a new batch. One other difference with kefir is that it contains as much as 1-2 % alcohol which gives it a kind of effervescence, but also helps the product last even longer than yogurt. I personally feel that kefir is a superior product to yogurt.

Acidophilus milk (*lactobacillus acidophilus*)

This product is milk to which acidophilus culture (beneficial bacteria) has been added. However, in this form, the milk is not actually cultured as yogurt. The milk is first ultra-pasteurized to reduce the other microbes. Acidophilus culture is then added. Acidophilus milk has the same culture as yogurt, but has not gone through the full thickening and culturing process. 26 In fact, contrary to what you might think, acidophilus milk actually imparts a rather sweet taste. Although you do not receive the same number of bacteria as you would from a cultured product you still receive some. I actually like this product and feel that it is a favorable food since the beneficial bacteria are delivered into the intestine where they will reproduce and deliver their positive results. Acidophilus can be purchased in capsules or powder from any health food store and added to various drinks as an extra source of beneficial bacteria.

Making cultured dairy products

Contrary to what you might think, it can be very simple to make your own cultured dairy products! Depending on which product you wish to make, establish your incubation location and temperature. You will need a thermometer and some type of incubator. In the past I have used the kitchen oven with just a 20-watt bulb as the heat source, or an inverted styrofoam cooler, or a heating pad with a pot over it ‾ (use your imagination.) The important point is that the temperature must be maintained ‾ if the milk gets too hot the bacteria will die, if too cold they will not reproduce. (The required temperatures are noted above.) You can also purchase a yogurt maker in most health food stores.

First, bear in mind that you must start with sterile milk! But rather than going through the scalding process as I describe above, you can begin with dry, powdered milk. Powdered milk as sold is basically a sterile product. I prefer the non-instant type, but either that or the instant varieties will do. Depending on the thickness of the end product you want, you add more powdered milk. If the instructions for mixing "milk" call for one cup of powder per quart, you add more; usually doubling the amount is about right, but experiment and judge for yourself. Here's the way to do it:

In a blender (or mixing bowl) start with warm water. Blend in your powdered milk, then blend in your starting culture. You can use fresh yogurt or acidophilus, or kefir. As an example, one or two tablespoons of fresh starter should be sufficient. Yogurt requires 4-6 hours, kefir requires about 24 hours. I have tried different combinations of starting cultures purchased from the health food store with interesting results. Bear in mind also that each of these products is easily contaminated with yeast and other airborne microbes, so keep them covered. If your end product begins to smell "yeasty" start your next batch with a new culture from the store.

DAIRY REFERENCES

1. Williams, RJ; Haffly,JD; Bode CW. "The Nutritive Value of Single Foods". National Academy of Science, April 28, 1971.
2.http://www.unu.edu/unupress/unupbooks/80338e/80338E00. htm
3. http://www.cce.cornell.edu/food/expfiles/topics/brenna/ brennaoverview.html
4.http://www.foodsci.uoguelph.ca/dairyedu/pasteurization. html

5. H.J. Heinz Company, Nutritional Data. Fourth Edition. 1960

6. Kutsky, Roman J. Handbook of Vitamins Minerals and Hormones. Second Edition. 1981.

7. http://www.nofamass.org/programs/rawmilk/index.php

8. http://www.gov.nf.ca/agric/pubfact/dairy/lsd005.htm

9. Keith Schneider. "FDA warns the Dairy Industry Not to Label Milk Hormone Free". New York Times, Feb. 8, 1994, p A1.

10 Michael K. Hansen, "Testimony before the Agriculture Committee of the Canadian Parliament on Potential Animal and Human Health Effects of rbGH Use by Michael K. Hansen, Ph.D.," dated March 9, 1994. Available from: Consumer Policy Institute, Consumers Union, 101 Truman Ave., Yonkers, NY 10703-1057. Telephone (914) 378-2000.

11 http://www.holisticmed.com/bgh/prostate.html

12 http://eagle.westnet.gr/~cgian/rbst.htm

13 http://home.intekom.com/tm_info/rw80917.htm

14 Lippman, Marc E. The development of biological therapies for breast cancer. Science, Vol. 259, January 29, 1993, pp. 631-32

15 Papa, Vincenzo, et al. Insulin-like growth factor-I receptors are overexpressed and predict a low risk in human breast cancer. Cancer Research, Vol. 53, 1993, pp. 3736-40

16 Stoll, B.A. Breast cancer: further metabolic-endocrine risk markers? British Journal of Cancer, Vol. 76, No. 12, 1997, pp. 1652-54

17 Brown, Ellen, JD, Hansen, Richard, DMD, FACAD, The Key To Ultimate Health, Advanced Health Research, Pub., CA, 2000.

18 http://asgsb.indstate.edu/programs/2003/72.html

19 http://www.meadowfresh.com/XO1.html

20 http://www.techno-preneur.net/timeis/technology/MaySciTech/DairyProduct.html

21 http://www.foodsci.uoguelph.ca/dairyedu/yogurt.html

22 European Journal of Clinical Nutrition (2002) 56, 843-849. doi:10.1038/sj.ejcn.1601399.

23 http://www.nature.com/ejcn/journal/v56/n9/abs/1601399a.html

24 http://muextension.missouri.edu/explore/hesguide/foodnut/gh1183.htm

25 http://www.midvalleyvu.com/Kefir.html

26   http://www.mycustompak.com/healthNotes/Food_Guide/Milk.htm

II.

SUBACUTE CLINICAL DEFICIENCIES

Abstract

*W*ouldn't *you like to know if indeed you are deficient of certain nutrients?*

Whether a clinician or a lay person, it sometimes becomes very helpful if nutrient deficiencies can be recognized by outward signs. This chapter will give you the more easily seen outward signs of several of the important nutrient deficiencies. The more you practice by looking at different subjects, the greater will become your proficiency at recognizing their deficiencies.

One of the most helpful things I've learned and used in clinical practice is the ability to recognize very subtle nutritional deficiency signs. By this I mean that there are some very simple ways to determine if a person is deficient in certain specific nutrients. You should understand that these "signs" are not the only problem that occurs during the deficiency of a nutrient. These are simply helpful ways to ascertain without expensive tests if indeed there might be a deficiency of that nutrient.

Some of these deficiency signs are rather simple to ascertain when you know what to look for. Unfortunately, there are only several nutrients that are recognizable. But let's go through them.

Vitamin A - Vitamin A is considered to be the nutrient that nourishes all epithelial tissue. Vitamin A as such, is only found in animals and animal products.1. Provitamin A also called collectively "carotenoids" are found in the plant kingdom and can be changed into vitamin A in the body. However, although vitamin A can be made from the carotenoids, the carotenoids cannot be made from vitamin A. Both are vitally important nutrients.

Epithelial tissue is "covering tissue"; tissue that covers and/or surrounds organs and other parts of the body. The skin, the largest organ of the body is epithelial tissue. The lining of your digestive tract from the mouth to the anus is epithelial tissue. In the same manner, the lining of your lungs and your entire respiratory system is lined with epithelial tissue. Each of your organs is covered with peritoneum, which also is epithelial tissue.

Hence the first place we look for in a vitamin A deficiency in the most obvious of these tissues, the skin. Medically, there is a condition known as "Keratosis Pilaris" This is described as a roughening of the skin, much like "gooseflesh". When you look closely, keratosis is expressed as a raising of the skin where the hair shaft is coming out from the surface. In some cases, you can actually see a coiled hair within the raised "bump". 2. 3. Also in some individuals there can be some pus within the raised "bump". The most common area for keratosis is on the back of the arms. It also can be found on the skin over the spine and rarely on the skin over the sternum or breastbone. Medically, this is treated with various topical medications, but taking orally encapsulated fish liver oil vitamin A easily clears up the condition. It is important however to understand that the results will take up to 3 months. This is because it takes at least that long for the body to make the changes in the skin itself. After that amount of time I have usually instructed my patients to take a good hot soaking bath and then to use a loofah sponge on the rough areas. This may have to be repeated several times in order to remove all of the roughness. It is equally important to know that if a vitamin A deficiency is obvious on the skin, it is also more than likely present in the other tissues mentioned above. Hence, the absorptive surfaces of your intestinal tract may not be functioning properly, thereby not allowing ideal absorption of nutrients.

Since the linings of the respiratory tract are also epithelial tissues, they are also affected by a vitamin A deficiency. This may be the cause of air borne allergens passing into the blood and acting as antigens causing allergies to certain air-borne particles. The same is true of the intestinal tract. If it is not properly nourished with vitamin A, there will be the possibility of what has recently been termed the "leaky gut syndrome". Because the cells of the gut or intestine are not properly in tact, partially digested materials can pass through into the blood stream also acting as allergens causing allergies.

Vitamin A is also known to enhance the resistance towards certain diseases. This is due, no doubt to the epithelial tissues offering a more intact barrier to the entrance of certain organisms into the body, especially within the lungs.

The second area to look for a vitamin A deficiency is in the eyes. In particular, in the whites of the eyes right at the "blink-line" on either side of the iris. That is where both the upper and lower lids touch. With a long-term vitamin A deficiency, a yellowish thickening will be seen in the white of the eyes at the blink-line. In advanced cases the results are a condition known as Bitot's spots, which again are a manifestation of an epithelial tissue problem caused by a vitamin A deficiency. Invariably, the thickened "sclera" will become yellowish as it worsens. This "thickened sclera" as well as Bitot's spots occurs only in long-term vitamin A deficiencies! 4. Where keratosis can develop in a relatively short time, such as 6-8 months, the eye-signs can take several years to develop. Knowing this, if a person has the eye-sign but not the keratosis, we can assume that he or she had a bad vitamin A deficiency some time in the past, but not now. Perhaps he/she is now on a better diet or taking supplementation. In contrast, if the person has keratosis but not the thickened sclera, we can assume that the deficiency has only been present for a relatively short duration. The question that many patients ask is can this problem be corrected? My answer is "yes" if one takes a natural supplement like fish liver oil. However, it will take several years to see the changes.

Vitamin B – The B vitamins work synergistically together. For that reason, even though different references give different symptoms for the separate B vitamins, I choose to consider each of the symptoms as a general vitamin B deficiency.

In general, a B vitamin deficiency can be manifested in several areas of the body but primarily in three areas, the heart, the gastrointestinal tract and the nervous system.

But these symptoms such as certain heart and neurological problems are usually caused by a severe vitamin B deficiency. Yet in my 40 years of active practice I have seen but one severe full-blown case of beri beri. Which I might say was totally missed by other practitioners but entirely relieved with vitamin B therapy.

Of the psychoneurosis, the following symptoms have been described:

"Instability, forgetfulness, difficulty in orderly thinking, vague fears, uneasiness, and the development of the ideas of persecution". But more important in the recognition of still minor, what we call "subclinical" deficiencies of this vitamin we can see the following:

Cheilosis – This is cracks and redness as the corners of the mouth on each side.5.

Inflammation of the tip and margin of the tongue. To recognize this sign one would have to do some comparisons with friends and relatives to get some idea of what "normal" is. Our tongues are literally covered with "papillae" or taste buds. Ordinarily, they should be of a specific size, recognizable as tiny projections on the tongue. In a vitamin B deficiency, these taste buds or papillae become red, enlarged and inflamed. This can be an indication of an early vitamin B deficiency. Secondary to this, if the deficiency is long lived, these papillae then "atrophy" or shrink. This then is recognizable as smooth, shiny marginal areas of the tongue where the papillae have simply disappeared. Of course, a B deficient red tongue would have to be differentiated from a tongue that has, as an example been scalded with a recent cup of hot coffee. But in order to get a more or less second opinion as to whether or not someone has a B vitamin deficiency we can go to the next "sign" of a B vitamin deficiency.5.

<u>**Injected sclera**</u> – This is another sign that we find in the eyes. When looking at the whites of the eyes, they should be clear white. In fact blue white. By "injected sclera" we mean that the whites of the eyes have visible, enlarged red blood vessels. I call them looking like "road maps". In medical terms, this would be "congested sclera". 5. This is rather easy to spot when you study the eyes of friends and relatives and make comparisons. Of course, there are degrees of the severity of this condition just like the other signs listed above.

Once again eyes can become "injected" or reddened from other causes. For example if a person is subjected to considerable dust or smoke in their immediate environment. Or if the person is wearing hard contact lenses. Each of these can cause injected sclera. Hence, one sign alone will not convince me that a person indeed does have a B vitamin deficiency. But if two or even three are present, it is almost certain.

<u>**Vitamin C and Proanthocyanidins**</u> – A very obvious and apparent sign is the inadvertent rupture of tiny capillaries under the skin causing smaller red blotches (petechial hemorrhages) or larger bruises (ecchymosis).

Let me explain first that all of our cells and tissues are held together by connective tissue called "collagen". This also includes the cells of our blood vessels, the arterioles and the tiny capillaries. If the connective tissue of these vessels is not able to hold together, they fracture allowing blood to ooze into the tissue spaces, causing the visible "bruise". 6. 7. This can be expected if and when we are obviously traumatized from an accident. This is not uncommon. However, if we commonly find these tiny hemorrhages and bruises under our skin, and can't even remember how they got there, we are dealing with a serious problem. For example, brushing against the corner of a table should not really fracture blood vessels.

Vitamin C has long been suspected to be important in the production of collagen because the ruptured vessels under the skin is a symptoms of scurvy, but studies have been inconsistent as to whether Vitamin C is the only factor involved. Recent new information has been coming to light that other "synergistic factors" are equally involved. The most important being factors called "proanthocyanidins". The foods that contain this factor are onions, legumes, red wine, parsley and bilberry (blueberries and huckleberries). But the most abundant source is found in grape seeds, and can be purchased as Grape Seed Extract.

Vitamin E – Much of what vitamin E does cannot be seen. As an anti oxidant, and needed for for sexual health and heart health, and so much more. But one thing that can be seen is called *keloids*. This is abnormal tissue growth at the sight of a scar. It is almost like the piling up of tissue upon tissue until the scare is an ugly lumpish disfigurement.8. Much has been written about keloids, but most has been ways to treat them with surgery and or topical creams. I have found in my practice that keloids can be prevented by having sufficient vitamin E in the diet at the time of healing of the scar.

Topical application of vitamin E after the keloid is formed can help, but taking vitamin E internally will speed the results considerably.

Zinc – This is a deficiency that can be easily spotted. It is recognized as white "flecks" in the fingernails. Knowing that a fingernail from root to tip will usually take about six months to grow, can give you an indication as to approximately when your diet did not include sufficient zinc. This will usually be apparent in several fingernails at the same distance from the root. A single white fleck on one nail alone, however is usually an injury to that nail or just an anomaly.

REFERENCES –
SUB ACUTE CLINICAL DEFICIENCIES

1. Roman J. Kutsky, Handbook of Vitamins Minerals and Hormones. Second Edition. Van Nostrand Reinhold Co. 1981 p.181-190

2. http://www.dermnetnz.org/dna.kerapil/kerapil.html

3. http://www.drgreene.com/21_84.html

4. H.J. Heinz Co. 4th Edition 1960 p.24

5. Op. Cit. H.J. Heinz Co. p.32

6. Galley P, Thiollet M. A double-blind, placebo-controlled trial of a new veno-active flavonoid fraction (S 5682) in the treatment of symptomatic capillary fragility. Int Angiol 1993;12:69–72.

7. Cox BD, Butterfield WJ. Vitamin C supplements and diabetic cutaneous capillary fragility. Br Med J 1975;3:205.

8. http://www.nlm.nih.gov/medlineplus/ency/article/000849.htm

12.

NUTRACEUTICALS, PHYTONUTRIENTS & PHYTOCHEMICALS

In recent years a new class of nutrients has being recognized it is called "phytonutrients". To date more than 12,000 of these factors have been identified. Not falling within the known categories of vitamins and minerals, phytonutrients are important nutrients found in their most concentrated amounts in many vegetables and fruits. In general they are responsible for their color, hue, scent and flavor. Although some are found in grains and seeds, they are most abundant in foods such as tomatoes, green tea, grapes, broccoli, parsley, spinach, garlic and many of the berries. This is by no means a complete list.

Their most important claim to fame lies in the fact that they are all potent antioxidants, and can neutralize free radicals. These are highly reactive chemical substances that can lead to premature aging and disease.

Phytonutrients have also been shown to enhance the immune system, enhance visual acuity, and some even play a role in preventing cancer. Some are anti-inflammatory, antithrombotic, anti bacterial and anti-viral. Some reduce cholesterol, relax and strengthen blood vessels. In other words, these are important additions to anyone's diet. Once again, they are found in highest concentrations in vegetables and fruit. 1.2.3.4.5.

Bilberry

This is a common berry found in many parts of the world and has been found to be extremely valuable with many pathologies especially conditions of the eye (ophthalmology). Its main factors are called anthocyanocydes (anthocyanin). They fall under the general category of the flavonoids. Within the United States they are called huckleberries, yet there are over 100 species with similar names throughout Europe. .Bilberry has been used as a medicinal herb since the 16th century.

Because of its affinity for the retina, it aids in night vision and was used during WW II by the RAF to improve the visual acuity of their pilots. It aids in quicker adjustment to darkness as well as faster restoration of sight after exposure to glare. It has been used in cases of macular degeneration, cataracts, retinitis pigmentosa and diabetic retinopathy as well as night blindness. Its used does not end there. It has also been found useful in connection with vascular and blood disorders and shows some positive effects in the treatment varicose veins, thrombosis and angina. It strengthens capillary walls by nourishing collagen (intercellular glue). It is a natural antioxidant and because it is a capillary vasodilator may help to lower blood pressure. It can also reduce platelet aggregation (the formation of clots). Because it contains a substance called glucoquinine, which has the ability to lower blood sugar it may help in diabetes. 6.7.8.

CoQ10 / (Ubiquinone)

Coenzyme Q10 is one of the unique factors discovered relatively recently that is of profound use in the body. Considered one of the two most important nutrients in and for the body (the other being vitamin C) it is literally found within every cell, with the highest concentrations found in the heart muscle and liver. But unlike vitamin C ubiquinone is manufactured within the cell, yet unfortunately its production within the body decreases with age.

Enzymes are organic catalysts, and a co enzyme helps to facilitate that particular enzyme. CoQ10 acts as a catalyst for countless reactions within the cell none the least, which is the release of energy. Unfortunately, Statin drugs like Lovacol, Lipitor and Mevacor inhibit the natural intercellular production of CoQ10. Therefore, CoQ10

may prove to be an invaluable supplement when taking these drugs

We have learned that oxidative processes on a cellular level in the body are one of the main reasons for aging. Co Q10 as a strong antioxidant could also prove to be invaluable for longevity . .

This substance has been found useful in cardiovascular disease, Parkinson's disease, high blood pressure, periodontal disease, male infertility and as an immune system enhancer. .9.10.11.12.13.14

Free radicals are molecules with an unpaired outer electron. Because of this trait, they can cause chain reactions thus damaging innumerable cells in the body. CoQ 10 is a vibrant free radical scavenger, which no doubt accounts for a multitude of its beneficial effects.

Garlic

Garlic is one of those rare herbs that have been used for centuries by many cultures for a multitude of reasons. Besides the mythical claims that it wards off vampires and evil spirits, it has been used throughout the ages for its health and healing qualities.

Were it not for the fact that it has lasted the test of time, one might call it a fad or a nostrum. However, because of its history I feel we can be assured that garlic does indeed contain some valuable health treasures.

Only recently with our growing knowledge of biochemistry are we beginning to recognize those powerful factors held within that humble bulb.

Some of the factors that have been isolated thus far are these:

Alliin; allicin; ajoene;

Some of the studies that have been done indicate that some of the effects of garlic may be to reduce blood cholesterol and help maintain the elasticity of blood vessels (which can help prevent high blood pressure). It discourages the growth of many harmful organisms such as bacteria, fungi and viruses, and disables dysentery-causing amoebas. Furthermore it is a powerful antioxidant that can neutralize very dangerous "free radicals" that have been implicated in tumor growth, atherosclerosis and aging. 15,16,17,18,19.

Cruciferous vegetables

Because of their amazing concentration of anti cancerous phytochemicals, although we have already mentioned them in our chapter on cancer I feel that we should reiterate them here. Within the entire vegetable kingdom there are no others that contain these potent anti cancer factors. We are speaking of course about cabbage, broccoli, brussel sprouts, and kale. The phytochemicals they contain are the following; glucosinolates, crambene, sulforaphane and indole-3-carbinole. These isothiocyanates as they are called are found only in the cruciferous vegetables. Even more exciting is the fact that broccoli sprouts contain 20 to 50 times more of the anti cancerous agent sulforaphane than is found in mature broccoli!. 20, 21, 22.

REFERENCES- PHYTONUTRIENTS

1.   www.nutritional-supplement-info.com/phytonutrients.html
2.   www.ars.usda.gov/is/AR/archive/dec99/stage1299.htm
3.   www.realtime.net/anr/phytonu.html
4.   www.nal.usda.gov/fnic/etext/000102.html
5.   www.newstarget.com/001505.html
6.   www.kcweb.com/herb/bilberry.htm
7.   www.mdsupport.org/library/bilberry.html
8.   www.stevenfoster.com/education/monograph/bilberry.html

9.   www.bodybuildingforyou.com/   health-supplements/
coenzyme-q10-benefits.htm.

10. www.nci.nih.gov/cancertopics/   pdq/cam/coenzymeQ10/
healthprofessional

11. www.thedoctorsdoctor.com/labtests/coq10.htm

12. www.chinese-school.netfirms.com/   coenzyme-q10-heart-
disease.html

13. www.faculty.washington.edu/~ely/JOM5.html

14. www.life.uiuc.edu/crofts/bioph354/complex_i.html

15. www.ahrq.gov/clinic/epcsums/garlicsum.htm

16. www.garlic-central.com/garlic-health.html

17. www.hhp.ufl.edu/faculty/pbird/keepingfit/ARTICLE/
GARLIC.HTM

18. www.uni-graz.at/~katzer/engl/Alli_sat.html

19. edis.ifas.ufl.edu/MV064

20. http://lpi.oregonstate.edu/infocenter/foods/cruciferous/

21. http://www.femalemuscle.com/nutrition/cruc_veg.html

22. www.aicr.org/site/PageServer?pagename=dc_foods_
cruciferous

23. http://www.hopkinsmedicine.org/press/1997/
SEPT/970903.HTM

13

CONCLUSION
SOME TIPS IN GETTING STARTED:

The purpose for this book has been to alert you to the fact that our stores and supermarkets hold a wide discrepancy of food qualities. From the worst junk and even dangerous foods to the widest variety of healthy foods, all is available. And the choice is yours to make.

Surely, it will be quite a challenge to embark on this health journey. But to take an example from our own experiences that my wife and I have reiterated over and over again. "It is easier (and cheaper) to take the care and time necessary to produce health in ourselves and our children than it is to disregard that care and deal with the consequences of a junk food lifestyle and its resultant poor health. You think about it, isn't it easier and cheaper to provide our children with a quality diet that will produce good health, rather then to deal day after day and night after night with a crying, feverish, sick child?

Once again, the choice is yours.

When you read our chapters on meat and dairy, vitamins and minerals and phytonutrients you find that the dangerous food is out there, but so are the quality foods.

You will find that there is a way to complement your diet with nutritional supplements and "super foods" that can create health as it has never been before in the history of mankind. Why not? Don't you deserve it?

On the other side of the ledger, remember that it is not the occasional indulgence that will cause you your health problems, it is your regular habits. What are your regular habits?

Too much coffee? too much sugar?, too many French fries? We all have some weaknesses. Don't let them get out of control!

The new health pyramid has some very important suggestions. How many fresh fruits and vegetables do you eat each day? Can you increase that number up to four or five?

Remember that it is these fruits and vegetables that contain the very important "phytonutrients".

Let's go through a list of things you can do to get started into your new, healthier lifestyle:

-When shopping try first to find your foods in the fresh food section, then go to the frozen foods, only then go to the canned and packaged foods.

-Second, avoid going shopping for food when you are hungry. If you do you will surely be tempted to buy unnecessary, impulse things.

-Third, don't waste your money or your health on negative foods.

-Fourth, keep those junk foods out of your home especially if you have children. Neither you nor they need the extra temptation to munch on the "junkies" between meals or while watching TV.

-Finally, become a label reader. After reading our chapter on "food additives", you should understand why the fewer additives, the better.

Meat – If you choose to eat meat, this is how to proceed; If you live in a rural area, there will most likely be a farmer that will sell you meat. Understand however that such a farmer would likely not be able to sell you meat by the pound or cut. They will sell you by the whole, half or quarter beef. Then either they or you will make arrangements with a facility to have it cut and wrapped. With such an arrangement, from a half or quarter beef you will have a variety of cuts such as steaks, roasts, chopped beef etc. To find such a farmer, you might ask around by word of mouth. You might call or go to the local feed and grain store frequented by the farming community. Ask if they know of such a local farmer or rancher. If you get several names, call each and ask thus:

"Do you sell beef? How do you sell it, by the half or quarter? Do you use any antibiotics in your feed? Do you use any growth hormones? If they do, ask if they will raise you a steer free from those, <u>and guarantee it</u>.

Do you work with a private facility for cutting/wrapping? How do you "finish a steer" pasture or grain? (beef grain fed for 30 –60 days will produce more tender meat, but it will contain a higher content of fat.) If the steer is fed strictly pasture prior to slaughter, you would want that steer to be "on the gain" at that time. In other words gaining weight.

True, it will not be as tender as grain fed but it will be leaner.

So you might say that it is a "toss-up". Meat from a grain fed steer will be more tender for steaks but will have more fat. If you prefer hamburger or pot roast then in my books, the leaner the better.

If you are looking for steaks the hindquarters offer the better cuts.

Finally, if half or quarter of a beef is too much for you, make arrangements with a friend to split it.

If you are far removed from the "country", there are many supermarkets that sell "organic meat". But to be on the safe side, question the manager and if necessary call the farm that produces it and ask the questions I have above. Remember, if you use meat, it is worth this additional trouble.

<u>Poultry</u> – In the same manner as above, if in a rural area, search for a farmer that produces "organic broilers". These will be 8 –10 weeks old and quite tender. But, they should be free from antibiotics and hormones. Most broiler producers raise their flocks indoors, but if you can find someone who raises broilers on pasture, outdoors, consider yourself lucky even if you pay more for them.

Eggs – Here you can run into considerable confusion if you don't know what to look for. Most laying flocks are kept in small cages with 1-2 birds in each cage.

Most cages are so low that they do not allow the hen to raise her head normally.

These cages are kept inside with the cages stacked on top of each other.

Sometimes the stacks are two, three or even four tiers high. The feed is brought into the long line of cages by an auger. The water comes through a trough. The bottom of the cage is slightly tilted so that when an egg is laid, it rolls to a side of the cage where it is picked up by an attendant. These birds never get out of that cage for their entire lives. They never see the sun. They get no exercise. They never come in contact with a rooster. (though hens do not need a rooster to lay eggs).

With that brief introduction, what should we look for in healthy eggs?

First, the hens must not have antibiotics or hormones in their feed or water.

They should be "free run" this means that they are not held in cages.

If they are allowed to run in free pasture, so much the better.

If possible, the eggs should be "fertile". This means that the hens should have access to a rooster. Fertile eggs remain fresher, longer, retaining total nutrients without refrigeration.

Catch phrases such as "naturally nested" have little meaning except to confuse.

"Organic vegetables and fruit" – Although I am very much in favor of so called organically grown foods, the term "organic is very confusing. To the consumer it means raised without chemical fertilizers or pesticides of any kind. To the scientist or chemist it means that the chemical structure of the food is" carbon based" That means either a carbon chain or carbon ring. But, petrochemicals, and many other agricultural chemicals and hormones are thus defined as "organic". I've seen many professors' stick up their noses at the organic farmers stating that they "don't even knows what they are talking about". But, we indeed know what we want, and what we don't want!

Let's talk further about organic products and farming. Remember in our chapter on vitamins and minerals I mention **that if a specific mineral is not in the soil and in a soluble state in that soil, it will not be in the plants that grow on it.**

Virtually all farming uses only three basic chemicals; nitrogen, phosphorus and potassium. With these three chemicals most crops will grow well and look good.

Let me elaborate further. In the soils of the Pacific Northwest, there is no selenium. That mineral is totally missing. No matter how you farm or organically garden, your produce will not contain that mineral, unless you intentionally add it to the soil as a part of your fertilization.

Most minerals are found naturally in most soils, but are not necessarily soluble for the plants to use them. Hence, it's almost as though they are not there. This is the case with most of America's farmland. Most of the soluble trace minerals have been depleted with years of farming, and not returned in fertilizers. But there is a solution to this dilemma. The solution is soil microorganisms. Soil microorganisms help break down the insoluble rock minerals, making them soluble and hence available to the plants.

But, then there is another problem. It is the caustic nature of the farm chemicals that are being used. Many of them literally destroy the microorganisms that could be helping us.

So, the question that must be asked is "how do we best increase and aid these microorganisms? The answer is manure, green manure, compost and crop residues plowed back into the soil.

I've seen so-called "organic vegetables" that look terrible! Somehow they have not been correctly fertilized, and they show it. Most of those organically grown vegetables and fruit are attacked by bugs and viruses because like the human condition, they have been poorly fed and they are weak and susceptible to attack and disease.

Let me introduce what is probably a new word for most of you "biodynamic farming"

This is a much broader concept introduced by a man named Rudolf Steiner many years ago. The idea is basically to balance not only the organic matter in the soil, but the mineral composition as well. The latter is done by the introduction of a complete ground rock mineral source from specific areas that contain a wide variety of minerals. These two things will create plants that will resist most bugs and diseases.

So, you see, there is a lot to be said about organically grown food, and indeed some serious misconceptions.

Finally I want you to know that in my lifetime alone there has been a tremendous improvement and availability of quality organic foods that were not available 30 or 40 years ago. The reason is because through education the demand for quality food has grown phenomenally. In our system, demand will result in supply. If the producers know there is a market for something, they will find a way to supply it.

Hence, if you still cannot find some of these quality foods, simply ask for them. If enough people do this, the supply will follow.

14.

BOWEL HEALTH

Abstract

*Y*ou've done it almost every day of you life, yet I'd venture to say
that most people have no understanding as to how the bowels
work and why bowel health is so important.

*Here we explain the mechanisms of the bowels and the forces that
cause them to move. We will find out that there are ways to improve
and strengthen bowel movements. We also will learn the dangers of
poor bowel function and how it can cause diverticulosis, polyps and
even cancer.*

Because of its importance, I have decided to include this
chapter in our book.

Although it actually begins before we are born, and
continues throughout life, most of us take the act of moving our
bowels more or less for granted. It's just something we "do." But
the significance of this process is vitally important if indeed we
want to achieve and maintain excellent health. From the early
days of my health education I can recall the statement by several
of the old-timers that "good health begins in the bowels." We
might also consider the corollary that "bad health begins in the
bowels." Let me explain how and why.

The digestive tract is, in simple terms, a "minor miracle." In
order to provide nutrients to the three trillion cells that make up

our bodies, the food that we eat must be processed and delivered to them via the bloodstream. Once the food is in the mouth, it is broken down physically by the teeth as well as chemically by several digestive enzymes in the saliva. The masticated food then proceeds to the stomach where it is further broken down physically by the "churning" of the stomach as well as chemically by the action of additional digestive enzymes.

Eventually in the small intestine, the bolus of food is totally broken down into the simplest components that can be readily absorbed into the body. As this bolus passes through the small intestine by the wave-like muscular contractions called "peristalsis," the nutrients are absorbed. Eventually that which remains unabsorbed within the digestive tube must be excreted from the body. This physical waste, called feces, passes into the large colon. The storage place for this waste is in that part of the large colon called the rectum. In severely constipated individuals, feces can accumulate into other parts of the large colon as well. Ideally, according to many health authorities, waste matter should be removed through bowel movement several times each day. Certainly at least once a day is vitally important! If this is not done, several serious problems can occur.

The large colon has within its wall very sensitive nerve endings. Unlike the nerve endings in your fingers that can detect heat, cold, pain, etc., the nerve endings in the rectum are sensitive to stretching. As the rectum fills with fecal matter, the bowel walls begin to stretch. This stretching sends nerve signals to the brain. The brain interprets the impulses as a filled and enlarged colon and sends other signals to the muscles in the bowel walls to begin contracting with wave-like peristaltic contractions. This triggers the urge to defecate.

It is important that this urge is acknowledged and the process completed. If this impulse to defecate is not fulfilled by a bowel movement at that time, and if this urge is continually sublimated, the nerve endings in the bowel will eventually loose their sensitivity. As this happens again and again, the bowels will require being filled to greater and greater capacity before the signal is finally sent to the brain for peristalsis to begin. You might say that the nerve endings become de-sensitized. This may cause the person to have longer and longer times between bowel movements because the bowels will need to be filled with increasingly greater quantities of feces before the signal for peristalsis and defecation is finally sent to the brain. This causes the feces to remain in the bowels for longer periods of time, which further exacerbates the problem.

If the fecal matter is not excreted within a reasonable time, it will loose moisture and begin to harden, making the next movement even more difficult. As the feces remain in the bowel, the digestive enzymes within it continue working on the remaining material, producing several harmful chemicals as well as gas. Not the least of these chemicals is a cancer causing substance called 3 methylcholanthrene.1 Since we know that this chemical is a potent carcinogen, and we know that it is formed in the feces, it is not beyond reason to suspect that pre-cancerous polyps and eventually cancer can result from too infrequent bowel movements.

When fecal matter remains within the bowel longer than it should, the production of gas through chemical reaction is inevitable. In an impacted colon, the gas has no place to go. As more gas is produced, the pressure forces outward in the direction of least resistance, which is the bowel wall. Weak parts of the bowel wall will then balloon outward, causing pockets called "diverticuli." These diverticuli in the colon wall will eventually fill with fecal matter, further complicating the situation of stagnant feces, resulting in gas and carcinogenic chemicals that can eventually become colon cancer. Both polyps and diverticuli are dangerous and more than likely the result of poor bowel habits.

You may not have recognized it as such, but the act of defecation **typically requires two forces.** First, the action of peristalsis within the bowel serves to push the food bolus downward. The second force is voluntary bearing-down causing an increase of inter-abdominal pressure in the area surrounding the colon. This pressure around the colon is the other force that causes the bowels to evacuate. Both of these factors contribute to a normal bowel movement.

It has been my supposition for years that as we tend to demand instant mashed potatoes, instant coffee, instant cash, etc., we also want instant defecation. This presents a problem. By immediately and always bearing down for a quick B.M., we eventually weaken the muscles of peristalsis through disuse atrophy to the point where they will not perform strongly. The premise "if you don't use it, you loose it" applies to these muscles as well as the others in the body. The process of defecation is one that should not be rushed, and the normal sequence of events should be as follows:

1. Wait for the urge to defecate.

2. Use some inter-abdominal pressure (bear down) only long enough to cause the anal sphincter to open and start the movement.

3. Once the movement starts, back off the inter-abdominal "bearing down" pressure and allow peristalsis to carry the movement as long as possible. This can be assisted by panting (as in natural childbirth) to keep from bearing down.

4 At the end of peristalsis, there may be a minimal bearing down to finish the movement.

I have found that as one practices this method, not only will the peristaltic muscles be strengthened, but also there will be fewer problems with hemorrhoids, for it is the persistent use of inter-abdominal pressure that is the main cause of hemorrhoids. By strengthening the action of the peristaltic muscles, we need use less inter-abdominal pressure.

To reiterate, the action of peristalsis is initiated by the stretching of the bowel wall. As the bowel fills, it causes nerve endings in the wall to stretch, triggering peristalsis. Disregarding the normal urge to defecate can weaken this neurological signaling. Hence, the full bowel does not cause normal peristalsis to begin when it should, thus necessitating more and more bearing down.

In cases of severe and lasting constipation, I encourage the use of colonics to clean out layers of hardened feces in the bowels. A colonic is a procedure similar to an enema whereby a trained operator introduces warm water into the bowels through the rectum, causing the water to go deep into the bowels. During this procedure the therapist can encourage peristalsis by molding and massaging the colon area of the abdomen in order to loosen the feces and to stimulate the neurological receptors in the bowel wall.

Once we understand the mechanisms of the bowels, it seems very obvious that the squatting position during defecation offers an advantage since while squatting, the front of the left thigh is definitely pressing on the descending colon and rectum. This in itself is an excellent stimulus to the neurological receptors in the full bowel. Some countries have as their toilets mere holes in the floor, where it is necessary to squat for defecation. There are even specialized toilets that we can purchase that will facilitate this position.

An exercise that can be used to stimulate peristalsis can be done as follows: assume a kneeling position on the floor, sit back on your heels, trunk erect. Place your right flat hand, thumb edge inward, over the left abdomen, between the lowest left rib and the pelvis, press deep into the abdomen using the left hand to assist. Then, flex the body forward, rolling around the hand and thumb until the fetal position is reached. Remain in that position for several minutes. Repeat if necessary. You can often feel the "gurgle" of peristalsis begin. This exercise squeezes the filled colon, causing the walls to stretch, thereby stimulating the "stretch reflex" which will induce peristalsis.

One final point is this: like other conditioned "reflexes" the bowels can also be trained to respond to conditioning. Similar to the famous Pavlov experiments, the bowel movement impulse can be conditioned. [In his experimental work with conditioning of dogs, Pavlov rang a bell, and then fed the dogs, rang the bell and fed the dogs. He continued this over several months, feeding the dogs only after ringing the bell. At the conclusion of the experiment, he rang the bell but didn't present food. They all began salivating nonetheless, thus demonstrating the power of conditioning.]

Obviously, the best conditioning for bowel movements is to try to move the bowels at the same time every day, or in relation to some other activity. Many people feel that the best time is right after meals. During meals, peristalsis is occurring in the entire digestive tract to naturally move the bolus of food. This also includes some peristalsis in the lower bowel. Some people have a bowel movement as soon as they arise in the morning. Others have a movement after some light exercise. The bowel movement follows some specific activity.

Some people feel the necessity to encourage bowel movements by the use of laxatives. Because we sometimes find ourselves in unusual circumstances because of travel, time changes and other untoward events, a laxative can be helpful because the danger of stool retention can be a greater danger than the use of the laxative. One must be careful, however, not to overuse them. My recommendation for an occasional laxative would be only herbal compounds. These can be obtained in any health food store. Continuous use of laxatives will establish poor bowel health as well as bowels that are reliant upon them for any bowel movements at all. Some laxatives can be downright dangerous if used regularly.

One final word on diet: there are some foods that are "bowel friendly" and some that are not. This depends upon the amount of fiber they contain. In understanding fiber, one should note that there are actually two types of fiber. These are "food fiber" also called "soluble fiber," and "crude fiber." The benefit of food fiber is bulk which helps to fill the bowel and to activate the stretch reflex. Crude fiber has a different function. Crude fiber by its very nature is rough and abrasive. Its action is to scour the walls of the colon and give a gentle irritation, which stimulates peristalsis.

Some of the highest fiber-containing foods are beans, peas and other legumes, including baked beans, split peas, lima beans and black beans Bran cereals and other grain and wheat products are high in fiber, especially of the crude type. Oats, in particular are especially good because they are high in both types of fiber.

Leading the list of foods that are low in fiber of any type would be meat. Hence a diet solely of meat would be a very poor bowel-friendly diet. This is no doubt the reason why high meat diets have been linked with bowel cancer.

Once again, I cannot stress enough the importance of maintaining good bowel health. Try using the procedures I have mentioned – slow down, don't rush. Use a conditioned reflex to help you. Use the exercises I have recommended, and if necessary find a reputable and experienced colonic operator.

REFERENCES BOWEL HEALTH

http://www.thewolfeclinic.com/newsletter0209.html

706961

Made in the USA